Hot, Healthy, Happy

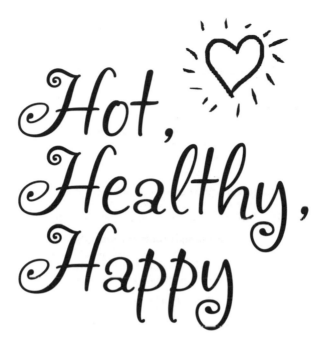

Hot, Healthy, Happy

The **21-Day Diet** to Eat, Drink and Think
Your Way to Self-Love and Skinny Jeans

Christy Fergusson PhD
THE FOOD PSYCHOLOGIST

HAY HOUSE

Carlsbad, California • New York City • London • Sydney
Johannesburg • Vancouver • Hong Kong • New Delhi

First published and distributed in the United Kingdom by:
Hay House UK Ltd, Astley House, 33 Notting Hill Gate, London W11 3JQ
Tel: +44 (0)20 3675 2450; Fax: +44 (0)20 3675 2451
www.hayhouse.co.uk

Published and distributed in the United States of America by:
Hay House, Inc., PO Box 5100, Carlsbad, CA 92018-5100
Tel: (1) 760 431 7695 or (800) 654 5126; Fax: (1) 760 431 6948 or (800) 650 5115
www.hayhouse.com

Published and distributed in Australia by:
Hay House Australia Ltd, 18/36 Ralph St, Alexandria NSW 2015
Tel: (61) 2 9669 4299; Fax: (61) 2 9669 4144
www.hayhouse.com.au

Published and distributed in the Republic of South Africa by:
Hay House SA (Pty), Ltd, PO Box 990, Witkoppen 2068
Tel/Fax: (27) 11 467 8904; www.hayhouse.co.za

Published and distributed in India by:
Hay House Publishers India, Muskaan Complex,
Plot No.3, B-2, Vasant Kunj, New Delhi – 110 070
Tel: (91) 11 4176 1620; Fax: (91) 11 4176 1630. www.hayhouse.co.in

Distributed in Canada by:
Raincoast, 9050 Shaughnessy St, Vancouver, BC V6P 6E5
Tel: (1) 604 323 7100; Fax: (1) 604 323 2600

Text © Dr. Christy Fergusson, 2013

A catalogue record for this book is available from the British Library.

ISBN 978-1-78180-082-9

Printed and bound in Great Britain by TJ International Ltd.

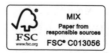

For Ella

Contents

Acknowledgments   *ix*

Introduction: Hello, Gorgeous!   xi

Part I: Hot, Healthy, Happy Beginnings

Chapter 1: Let's Get Personal   3

Chapter 2: What They Don't Want You to Know   11

Part II: Hot, Healthy, Happy Body

Chapter 1: Eat Yourself Skinny   19

Chapter 2: Eat Yourself Happy: Turning Dark Moods
                Technicolor   37

Chapter 3: Do You Have the Guts to be Healthy?   51

Chapter 4: Hormonal Havoc: Managing Your
                Monthly Madness   63

Chapter 5: Beat Breakouts: The Formula for
                Supermodel Skin   79

Part III: Hot, Healthy, Happy Mind

Chapter 1: Think Yourself Hot, Healthy, Happy   93

Chapter 2: Go With the Flow: How to Float Through
Life With Ease   103

Chapter 3: Growing Up Unprotected: How to Build
Strong Boundaries   115

Chapter 4: Your Inner Three-year-old: How to Heal
the Child Inside   127

Chapter 5: Dream Big: How to Get Anything You Want   139

Part IV: Hot, Healthy, Happy Life: The HHH 21-day Diet

Chapter 1: Ingredients for a Hot, Healthy, Happy Life   153

Chapter 2: Getting Started   171

Chapter 3: Transition to Hot, Healthy, Happy   191

Chapter 4: 21 Days to Hot, Healthy, Happy   199

Chapter 5: Hot, Healthy, Happy Recipes   243

Final Farewell: Hot, Healthy, Happy Ever After   265

Endnotes   267

Index   278

Acknowledgments

First, I'd like to thank my gorgeous husband, Jonathan, for all his love and encouragement. Thank you for making me green juice every morning and calming the chaos around me so I had time to write. I think we make a pretty great team.

When I feared I would never recover, my parents told me that no matter what, they would take care of me. Thank you both for your unconditional love throughout the years, and for always championing my dreams. I couldn't have done any of this without you both.

To Janie, if I could bottle your energy and give it to readers this would undoubtedly be a bestseller; thank you for all your support over the last few years, and to John for all the Friday night dinners.

I wish to say a huge thank you to all the clients I have worked with over the years – you have given me invaluable insights and experiences that have been instrumental in the creation of this book.

I would like to thank Carolyn Thorne for asking me to write, and for all her time and guidance over the past year. To Leigh Fergus for throwing my name in the hat, Amy Kiberd, and all the staff at Hay House UK who have been involved in this book.

I would like to give a big thank you to Sandy Draper for her fantastic job at editing; your ideas have been invaluable.

Gladys, thank you for clearing the clutter so I could think straight. You are an angel in disguise.

I would also like to thank Lawrence Scott for his brilliant photographs on both the book cover and throughout our website.

Finally, to my wild and insanely beautiful daughter, Miss Ella Summer White, thank you for reminding me how to play, laugh at silly stuff, and dance like a banshee. I hope the words we say at night will one day help you to manifest your dreams. 'I am loved. I am healthy. I am happy. I am going to do great things in this world.' I don't doubt it for a second, sweetheart.

Introduction
Hello, Gorgeous!

Here we are.

You have your face buried in another diet book and I have a story to tell.

Before we begin, I have a little confession. This isn't your typical diet book. There are a million ways to lose weight, countless formulas for skinny, but that's not what you're really after, is it? Sure, a perfect-size waist would be awesome, and who would knock having a tight tush and feeling great in their skinny jeans, but looking and feeling hot requires much more. You may be fed up with feeling overweight but what about your skin? Does it glow? Your digestive system, is it calm and content or crazy and clogged? Are your hormones happy or haywire?

Let's do some emotional arithmetic. What if you forgot overwhelm and instead just did things a little differently today than yesterday? You know, eat more goodness, move more, and think happier? How would tomorrow change? What if you chose to stop hiding? Hiding behind the status quo, fear of failure, and negative thinking? What if you didn't pay your money at the crazy, diet-town tollbooth and forgot all about calories, fat grams, and food obsessions? What would life look like then?

Your springboard to skinny jeans and self-love has arrived

You're here. You've showed up, opened the page at something different, and I'm psyched to go on this journey with you. So leave those old records – 'I have no commitment,' 'I don't have enough time,' 'Nothing I do ever works' – behind and plug in to your power. Give your body and soul a makeover. Declare your superpowers. Stop snorting stress, getting high on jellybeans, and start living life on your terms. Let's get your body smiling. Polish that inner and outer shine. Crowd-surf our way to stunning and dive into the messy beauty of you.

This book is a nutritional, psychological, and spiritual toolkit to becoming hot, healthy, and happy in the modern world. Consider this your official invitation to the life and body you want. *Psst... the sooner you RSVP the better.*

If you feel stuck I sympathize because I've been there. Not long ago I was overweight and chronically ill: disastrous digestion, hormone havoc, and acne attacks. I spent years obsessing over calories, throwing up in bathrooms, and starving. I was lost. My wake-up call meant lifestyle overhaul 101. I met my inner hot, healthy, happy heroine and reconnected with my body: *Hey gorgeous, where have you been!* The myriad of physical symptoms packed their bags, taking the body hang-ups and food issues with them. I stopped weighing food, counting calories, points, and fat grams, and got skinny and healthy in mind and body. I learned some incredible things along the way, and I'm going to share my treasure trove of goodies with you here.

Going back is the way forward

We're going to go back to a time when things were simpler. Before your dinner became a multibillion industry and before

TV advertisements, nutritional pyramids, and crisp white coats dictated how and what you ate. It's time to be a trailblazer: a savvy girl who knows her body and mind.

I'm going to show you that science makes you sexy. How understanding your beautiful biochemistry makes you red hot and is far more reliable than any quick-fix diet or praying for a miracle. Once you master it you'll be able to decode your body and reprogram for a more vibrant you. You'll discover that health is more than simply the absence of disease or dysfunction: it's the glow of radiance. Health is free from blockages: it's living in a serene way, giving you harmony inside and out. It's incredibly simple, too: dump the junk and tune in to what your body and mind needs. It's time to bring all of you to the party.

First I want to redefine 'hot,' because it isn't about being the next top supermodel. Hot is about finding your inner mojo and waking up every day feeling super-psyched about being you. Forget fitting in, looking like everyone else, and being the same as your friends – they have that covered. But there is no one as good at being you as you. No one can steal your glitter when you're hot, healthy, happy. When you reach that place it is like an avalanche.

So what makes the HHH approach special?

The real reason is that this is one of the few programs out there that recognizes you're completely and utterly unique. Most diet books treat you as if you're just the same as everyone else. They teach you cookie-cutter programs which force you to ignore what your body needs, desires, and wants. Here, you'll find all the information you need to make up your own mind about what your body does or doesn't need; discover how to create a diet that suits you; and make informed decisions about what foods you put in your shopping basket, your body, and your mind.

☀ *Hot, Healthy, Happy: Do what feels right for you*

If, like me, you're a bit of a geek in disguise and want all the in-depth juicy details, then you'll get them because this book is packed to the gunnels with information and advice. But remember, we're leaving overwhelm at the door, and so I've given all the stuff that you *need to know* in HHH bite-sized panels, just like this one. So watch out for these but stay chilled and let yourself marinade in them for a while. Then relish selecting what suits your lifestyle from the health-crazed pick-n-mix on offer: do what feels right for you and leave the rest. Don't let anyone fool you into thinking that they know more about what your body needs than your body does. For that reason no expert on the planet knows how to make you healthy, happy, and hot better than you.

You are amazing. Don't believe me? Well, look at your hand for a second. Now scratch your nose. Nothing man-made comes close to the genius and complexity of everything it took for your body to do just that. You see your body already knows how to make, create, and manifest everything you want in your life; you just need to learn how to get out of its way. You and you alone are the creator of your health. That delicious individual staring back at you every morning in the mirror is exactly who you have manifested. Every choice, big or small, up until this moment has determined who you are, how you look, how you feel, and everything in your life.

Disempowered? Fed up? Just plain, old-fashioned tuckered out? Don't worry, you're only human and you're not alone. No one feels 100 percent all of the time. Everyone gets stuck knee-deep in life's sludge from time to time. However, it is precisely these times when you need to up the ante. The universe is constantly expanding and so are you: growing, grooving, learning, and evolving. That's non-negotiable. You are truly and utterly incredible. Yes, even those wobbly bits you're pinching with your fingers.

How do I know this when I haven't met you? I know because your body's cells are constantly regenerating. In seven years you'll be a completely brand spanking new you. Here's another thing: we all share 99.9 percent of the same DNA. Bet you didn't realize you had 99.9 percent of the same genetics as a supermodel. *Yeah, my 5ft 2in ass was shocked, too!* This means you have the capability to be whoever or whatever you want. We all have the wild rock star, Olympic athlete, creative artist, fabulous author, cool parent, spiritual healer, even super-sexy pop star gene just waiting to be expressed. Our genes don't hold us back from anything. In other words, whatever your health up to this point, whatever problems you're facing, you can overcome them and create a healthier you. Everything we need is right there waiting for us in our DNA.

But here's the important bit: what we eat, drink, and think changes how our genes react; they literally shape who we become day by day. You're in the driving seat. You create you. *Um yeah... you're that incredible.* Did you know you had that much power?

So the million-dollar question is, who do you want to be? Because here's the thing, you get to decide. Change now. Live now. Be happy now. Seize your life. Radiate. Manifest magic. Don't hang around waiting for others to give you permission, because they won't. I have your goddess of permission on speed dial and she is saying, get going. This is your time to shine.

That is what the HHH program is about. I'm not going to tell you what to do, I am going to give you all the information you need, and teach you to listen to what your body is asking for, how to intuitively understand what it is saying, and how to give it what it needs.

Here's how we roll *(spoiler alert):*

Part I: Let's get personal. I'll reveal the crazy road that got me here, but also the one thing that changed my relationship with food forever. If you want to free yourself from a lifetime of dieting torture then listen up.

Part II: Get informed about food and learn to speak your body's language so you can give it what it really needs to be hot, healthy, happy.

Part III: We'll dive deep into the pandemonium of the mind, your inner world, to learn the secrets of magnetic attraction.

Part IV: Here you'll find all the ingredients of a hot, healthy, happy life and they will start working immediately. All you'll need to do is stock up on your secret weapons and then follow my 21-day diet to eat, drink, and think your way to the body and life you want.

Pick up hot stuff

I've seen eye-popping transformations, not just in myself but in countless others who have used this process to shift their lives 180 degrees. Since changing what I eat, how I think, and how I live each day, my mind and body has been strong, focused, and at peace. From my early experiments on myself to my formal training as a nutritionist and psychologist, and my later work with clients, I have proved time and time again that this system works. Now it's your chance in the spotlight. Start the road less traveled to become your own hot, healthy, happy heroine.

As you make your way through this book, let go of what has come before and start afresh. A beginner's mind is an open mind. Think of each piece of new information as if it were a power seed being planted in the rich compost of your consciousness. Over time these seeds will grow and shape your life. The universe is always expanding and so are you. You change, grow, and progress all the time. By staying open these seeds will help you grow toward that fabulous, disco-dancing diva: shining in the spotlight and living every day like it's your last... new you.

And it's all beginning just over the page...

Part I
Hot, Healthy, Happy Beginnings

Chapter 1
Let's Get Personal

Most teenage girls collect handbags and shoes, but not me. Growing up, I collected diagnostic labels: endometriosis, polycystic ovarian syndrome (PCOS), dysmenorrhea, food intolerances, menorrhagia, candida, bulimia, migraines, insomnia, acne, irritable bowel syndrome (IBS), depression, myalgic encephalomyelitis (ME), and seasonal affective disorder (SAD). Forget liplocking with boys, underage drinking, and parties, because I had hot dates with my doctor, medications to swig, and dressed to impress for blood tests. While my friends were learning about science, I was living it; while they were shopping for makeup, I was stocking up on therapists, hypnotherapists, counselors, psychologists, herbalists, nutritionists, acupuncturists, naturopaths, reflexologists, and homeopaths.

You see, by the age of 12 I had chronic fatigue syndrome (CFS). I know that sounds like I was making it up, but after a year of feeling sick and tired (literally), and being dragged back and forth to the doctor, I was happy to take any label or prescribed medication a white coat would give me if it meant that life would resemble 'normality' again. I still recall the workings of my 12-year-old brain. Thought one: *Did it really take a year of me complaining about fatigue to come up with chronic fatigue? What are these guys doing at medical school?* Thought two: *Great, pass me the pills, let's get the show back on the road.* That's how it worked. Didn't it? Get sick, doctor gives diagnosis, throw back a pill: *Goodbye bed, hello world.* Whoa! Imagine if it were that simple. You certainly wouldn't be reading this book right now, and my life might have taken me in a completely different direction.

Human Rubik's Cube

Throughout my teenage years my body was the Rubik's Cube that wouldn't line back up. My teenage hormones were outraged, and I was frustrated with my inability to be like everyone else: *Why am I sick while everyone else is partying?* I didn't deserve this. I was a good girl: polite (sometimes), and I didn't shoplift or car jack. I was active. I even ate fruit and veggies, for heaven's sake. They should have been my wild rebellious years and I couldn't even get out of bed.

At school I was stigmatized. It's hard to be Little Miss Popular when you only show your face once a week; you miss parties, and even my teachers began to think I was skipping school. To summarize this very painful part of my life: my teen years weren't about essays and boys, they were spent traveling around the country meeting doctors and alternative therapists, brainwave devices, sunlamps, odd-tasting drinks, flower remedies, crystals, and frustrations. The medical profession just kept coming up with more labels and more quick fixes, but none of them worked. So, after four years of waiting for a miracle cure, I knew if I wanted a long-term solution that I'd have to figure one out for myself.

Stress head to detox junkie

Aged sweet 16, I was a girl on a mission: think Lara Croft with a bad headache. I put on my big-girl shoes and started figuring out why I was so sick.

The result? I spring cleaned my collection and restocked with something new: qualifications. The years that followed were spent with my nose in books. I trained for nine years to become a Doctor of Psychology and Chartered Psychologist, another four years as a Nutritional Therapist specializing in Functional Medicine, and finally undertook a year's training in Clinical Hypnotherapy. In a nutshell, a PhD, MSc, BSC (Hons.), BA (Hons.), Diploma, and Chartership. *Slacker. Eh?*

While studying hard I also began compiling a laundry list of my health complaints. I figured my hormones were haywire. Why? Because most months were spent scrunched in a ball under the bedcovers. Surely that wasn't right? My acne was soul destroying, my gut had road rage, my joints ached like a senior citizen's, my eyesight was shot, and Prozac was my new best friend. If I were going to leave these health issues behind, I knew my life needed a makeover. It obviously wasn't going to be simple, but a twinge of hope had been sparked. Maybe I could figure this out after all?

I was 19 when I discovered a health food shop. Don't take that lightly – I come from Scotland, home of the deep-fried Mars bar. I found myself there on a dark, rainy day – *they're all like that in Glasgow* – clutching a piece of paper with the words take out wheat, dairy, sugar, and caffeine on it. Sounded easy enough. It was only four things after all. How hard could it be? Well, as it happened, my local grocery store *reeaaally* loved all those things. In fact so much so, they were in almost everything I usually ate, apart from the odd fruit or vegetable.

I was bewildered. These foods weren't advertised on the TV, that was for sure. The packaging was weird. The prices? *An organic cucumber costs how much?* Nevertheless, I raced around the store, throwing green leafy foods, odd-looking jars, books, supplements, and powders into my basket: *What were Kale chips, spirulina, chlorella, hijiki, and quinoa?* For a girl living on chocolate-spread sandwiches, low-calorie microwave meals, and packet noodles this was a whole new existence. This wasn't just a diet makeover, as I was catapulted into the world of cleansing and detoxification. Overnight I went from a food-addicted stress head to a detox junkie. I traded my diet drinks for veggie juices and my fake tan for skin brushing. My parents feared I'd joined a cult.

I wish I could say I juiced that pricey cucumber and, abracadabra, I was cured. But life isn't the movies and you're only in Chapter 1, so you may have guessed there's more to this tale. Stubborn symptoms persisted and my body still wasn't 100 percent convinced. In my head I had it all figured out, but my skin wasn't playing ball, my hormones were temperamental, and I was still hung up on food. Then my 20s rolled round and I fell in love... and it wasn't with a hunk or pill-shaped.

Divine balance

I discovered functional medicine, and boy did it rock my world. *Ta dah! Not impressed? Well listen up and you will be.* Functional medicine works by treating the body as an integrated system, and I realized that all my symptoms were like a spider's web – *inter-freaking-connected.* For me it was a health revolution because, by testing to pinpoint exactly where the imbalances lay, I was able to say goodbye to the abundance of medically prescribed labels, the million daily pills, the supplements, the powders, and the disgusting concoctions. I finally knew precisely what to take. So that year I stopped asking for jewelry for my birthday and clothes at Christmas. Instead I asked for private lab tests. The cult just got a little pricier. Nonetheless I started getting answers.

💡 Understanding functional medicine

Functional medicine aims to address the underlying cause of disease stemming from our lifestyle choices, any environmental exposure, and our genes. It focuses on creating moments of deep insight into the mind, body, and spirit which provide in-depth answers to complex and often stubborn health issues. Visiting a functional medicine practitioner usually involves an in-depth case history consultation, the completion of questionnaires, and undergoing laboratory testing. The information gathered is then used to assess the underlying imbalances and influences (genetic, environmental, or psychosocial) that have created the context for the condition or symptoms. Based on this, a customized treatment plan is developed to rebalance the system and restore health.[1]

So you could say I became my own human guinea pig. No ethics committee needed, just a sprinkle of hope and a whole lot of guts. Somewhere in my journey I discovered my own hot, healthy, happy healer. She was intuitive, strong and didn't take any nonsense. And what I learned I'll be sharing with you in this book, so don't worry, they'll be no pinpricking involved... not unless it's something that appeals, of course.

What I discovered transformed my health, my body, and my outlook. As you'll find out soon enough, as each imbalance is restored to health, others vanish. It is a super health, disco-domino effect: skin healing, digestion divine, and energy levels ignited. The crazy part? The excess weight starts freefalling off without a whisper of calories, fat grams, portion sizes, or starving. I know this is true because I transformed into the enigma I had mud-wrestled for years: a skinny chick who eats the food she loves. *I know, I thought it was an urban myth, too!* Turns out science does make you sexy after all.

- -

☼ *Hot, Healthy, Happy: The best prescription in the world*

♥ **Stop** focusing on illness; focus on health.

♥ **Listen** to your body when it speaks.

♥ **Treat** yourself with love.

♥ **Stop** defining health by diagnostic labels assigned by the medical profession.

- -

What's your muse?

Think about it... what made you pick up this book? What is stopping you from being hot, healthy, happy?

♥ Excess weight?

♥ The blues?

♥ Hormonal chaos?

♥ Digestive troubles?

♥ Low energy?

♥ Poor skin?

♥ All of the above?

If so, then the HHH 21-day diet could be your savior.

And what about your head? What you put in to that counts too, you know. How about guilt, regret, sadness, or a heart-wrenching breakup? It doesn't matter what it is, it's how you respond that counts. Make it your catalyst for transformation, your muse not your captor. It's time to take back control and give your body and soul a vitality makeover.

For years I believed that knowing how to take care of my body was like trying to solve a mammoth Sudoku brain-teaser: impossible. So-called experts held me health hostage. It doesn't need to be that way. After all, aren't humans designed to be healthy? Strip away the unhelpful labels you've assigned and stop getting in the body's way. Let's demystify the process and make you the expert, the guru, the game changer. That's the only way you'll ever become hot, healthy, happy. Once you're in the know, those quick fixes, gimmicks, and miracle cures will lose their shimmer.

The great thing is that, unlike me, you don't need to wait until your body is falling apart. Take action now. Listen to your body, throw out the bathroom scales *(yes, I mean that!)*, the marketer's mantras, and scratch the words, calories, food points, and fat grams from your vocabulary. Start talking your body's language. If you're feeling off kilter then discover what your body is trying to tell you. Think of your symptoms as being Morse code from the body – it's trying to tell you something. If you're not feeling like a rock star then you need to start listening to your body's SOS call.

If you want to wear those skinny jeans with pride then get healthy. If you get healthy, you'll get skinny. That's right. The diet industry has us so distracted that we miss the real, long-term solution: your body already knows how to be slim. You just need to tune in, dig deep, and find the root cause of the imbalances.

So this book is my love note to you. Inspired by my difficult journey from that dark alleyway in my life to a place of health, delicious foods, and glorious sunshine. At rock bottom I mined and came up with gems. My ill health forced me to rethink how I saw my body and begin to work in cahoots with it instead of against it. This book contains years of my research and work with clients, and I've packed it to the gunnels with the transformational information I've learned and seen work miracles time after time.

Are you ready to meet your hot, healthy, happy healer? This woman is going to supercharge your life. Forget obsessing over niggling symptoms and hunting down miracle pill-popping cures. Let's do the work and start making changes.

Chapter 2

What They Don't Want You To Know

Let me be honest, I love modern-day living. Instant chat over more than 100,000 miles. *Awesome.* Drunken celebrity tweets direct to your phone. *Hilarious.* But with new advances have come misuse and confusion. We can power up an iPad, but what about kick-starting our bodies? We can rule technology, but have we lost touch with ourselves? Many moons ago, before we could Facebook stalk our exes and technology streamlined the way for convenience, we ate real food. We didn't need dieticians, magazines, scientists, journalists, or big corporations telling us what we *should* be eating. We trusted our inborn wisdom rather than our calorie intake, low-fat labels, or food points.

As the years went by things changed. The earth, trees, and oceans aren't the only places food comes from now. We no longer grow and catch it ourselves. Instead, food comes out of packets, tubes with smiley characters, plastic containers, the freezer, and via the drive-thru window. Foods now have faces and personalities. The poor fresh foods have become uncool next to the new kids on the block with their shiny packages, fluorescent colors, and amazing textures. Bold and confident, if the real foods could speak you would hear them shouting: 'Throw me in your basket, I'm made with whole grains,' 'I'm high in fiber, and fortified with B vitamins,' 'Drink me, I'm full of good probiotic bacteria, your digestive system will love me,' 'Leave that diet stuff, pick me, I'm naturally low in fat and sugar. I'll make you skinny and gorgeous just like that girl in the advert... you deserve to be popular, sexy and fun, too.' Overnight our dinner has become a multibillion industry involving focus groups, catchphrases, branding, and subliminal messages.

Nowadays large corporations control our food and bankroll grocery-store hotspots. We have fallen head over heels for the tastes, the promises, and the belief that these foods will transform our lives. They study how we think, what makes us tick, and how to make us go gaga for their products. Nowhere is safe: TV, radio, billboards, magazines, grocery stores – everywhere we look we are being conditioned to drug ourselves up with food. Forget real food, we are eating 'food-like products' jazzed up to make them incredibly moreish.

Clever advertising sells us fantasyland. Manufacturers whisper sweet promises, like the bad-boy player who promises to stay faithful then runs off with your best friend. Your mind is a sophisticated, hi-tech computer. Forget whiz-kid software and smart phones, your brain's abilities could blow them out of the water. Marketers are the computer geeks of our minds. Their livelihoods depend on figuring us out. How many people take the time to learn how the mind works? Usually we're too busy tweeting. But here's the thing, the more you avoid learning how to change your thoughts about food, the longer you'll stay stuck.

Is your biochemistry screaming BS?

It's not just our minds being whacked out of sync. Food manufacturers also use our biochemistry against us. *How rude!* Our beautiful genes have become their weapon. The very programming that once helped us survive is now making us ill. As we are naturally inclined to seek sweet tastes, fat, and salt, the multibillion corporations have super-charged their products to appeal to our instincts, and these ramped-up sweet, fatty, and salty foods have caught us hook, line, and sinker. It's a double whammy.

Think about your typical soft drink advert. You see some goddess-like creature swigging back a can of pop while topping up her tan. The little voice in your head whispers: *That could be me if I drank that.* The truth is you're being duped. Reality check, here's what's not on the label: this drink contains phosphoric acid that leaches your body of essential minerals (e.g. calcium[1]), artificial sweeteners that will make you fat[2] (more on that shortly), or high fructose corn syrup that will increase your risk of diabetes.[3] Just for your extra pleasure we have added a dangerous cocktail of aspartame and caffeine. This powerful excitotoxin is guaranteed to give you a little buzz as it kills off some of your brain cells,[4] and that's why nothing quite hits the spot like a... [*add your brand of poison here*].

☀ *Hot, Healthy, Happy: Make informed choices*

Which would you choose: low-fat granola bar or avocado? Don't be fooled. Real foods and food-like products are worlds apart. Most fat phobes would grab the granola bar over the avocado. However, our beautiful biochemistry is calling BS. Your body knows exactly what to do with the delicious good fats in the avocado: how to break them down and extract all their goodness. The nutrient-devoid, sugar-packed granola bar is about as much use to your body as eating a wooden spoon. Pass me the avocado any day. Being hot, healthy, happy is about making informed choices about what you eat.

Healthy eating meltdown

We live in healthy eating overload mode. Foods are nutritional jigsaw puzzles and scientists our modern-day farmers. We don't talk food anymore – *that's so last season* – nutrients are the new 'in' thing. We no longer see the wood for the trees, or the berries from the flavonoids. Real, whole, natural foods have become yesterday's news. Instead it's all about phytochemicals, antioxidants, carbohydrates, proteins, and a whole list of complicated words we really don't need to know. Why waste time eating carrots when we can just pop a beta-carotene supplement? The thing is, it's the synergy within the whole food that our body needs. If I were to cut down the heels of your new stilettos, would they still be as awesome? No way! Sometimes things should just be left as they are: your food and your killer heels!

Eating should be instinctual, not make you want to pull your hair out. As a result of unnatural ways of living, we've lost touch with our natural intuition around food. Our groovy survival instinct has been tinkered with and our system is in self-destruct mode. Autoimmune diseases, heart disease, the big C, type 2 diabetes, and obesity are raging out of control. We are stuffing our faces, starving ourselves, obsessing about food, throwing it up. It's beyond nuts. We are physically and emotionally pretzeled.

JUST TELL ME WHAT TO EAT! How many meals should I have? What size is a portion? What percentage of fat do I need? Suddenly we need a degree in nutrition just to know what to throw in our shopping baskets. Thank heavens for the trusted 'experts' with their pyramids, charts, and shopping lists of manufactured foods. How could we get through dinner without them? We turn to slimming clubs, magazines, fad diets, and even the surgeon's knife. We are screaming inside for someone to take control of our eating because we've lost touch with what we need. We have more diets now than actual real foods. One minute low fat is 'in,' then high protein, then low carb, then counting calories. Being slim and healthy has become a mathematical equation. Dinner plates look more like pie charts than eating implements. Our survival GPS, which kept us alive for millions of years, has been overloaded and is in desperate need of a reboot.

Breaking the rules

It's time to grab back the reins and become the CEO of your mind and body. Forget calories, fat grams, points, and all the other dieting white noise. It's time to start breaking the 'rules.' Gorgeous models, expensive advertising, and branding may be able to trick your mind into thinking some foods are good for you, but your body doesn't lie. If you're depressed, overweight, tired, hormonal, or constipated then your body is hollering for help. It's time to answer its call. Recharge your mojo. Are you ready to throw away the marketers 'I'll-make-you-beautiful' tinted glasses and watch your inner goddess strut past the smoke and mirrors? Let's rewire your mind and body for creativity, personal responsibility, individuality, and human connectivity, and get doped up together on self-love. Think of the information to come as your Swiss army knife for being hot, healthy, happy in the modern-day world.

The truth is there are many things in life you can't control – traffic, blizzards, string bikinis, and hot pants – but you're the star commander of your health and happiness, and it is all to do with what you eat, drink, and think. What you choose to feed yourself physically and psychologically is vital. That is why *Hot, Healthy, Happy* is much more than a 21-day diet. It is a process of discovery that will 'hook you up' to your inner wisdom. Get ready, your body's about to go on speakerphone.

Part II
Hot, Healthy, Happy Body

Chapter 1
Eat Yourself Skinny

It's confession time again. I was once a diet addict. Definition of insanity: doing the same thing over and over again and expecting different results. I deserved a straitjacket because no matter how many miracle plans failed, I hopped onto that dieting treadmill again and again. Surely there had to be a secret formula to skinny. How else could you explain a size zero or supermodel collarbones? So a bookcase of diet books later, did I find a magic formula? Yes, I did... not one but hundreds. The problem? They involved following so-called formulas. You know, counting and such nonsense. *Go figure*.

Let's be serious. No one wants to have to do arithmetic just to eat breakfast, but there I was, weighing, calculating percentages, counting points, charting, and measuring. Every system had different rules. I was high protein all day till the munchies hit, then I was jamming the high-carb plan splayed out in front of the TV. It was a diet mix 'n' match disaster.

Years of yo-yo dieting passed, until one day I'd had enough. I decided to create my own foolproof dieting system. Nothing fancy, no counting and with only two rules. I had surpassed myself.

Rule one: eat as little as humanly possible. Rule two: when the moment takes you, eat the entire fridge contents and throw it up. Simple. Why was no one else trying this? *Er, yeah, Christy it's called bulimia.* So for a while I lived on 350 calories a day, pretending to eat, throwing up, and measuring my thighs and waist daily. My winning number was 7st 7lbs (47.5kg). Heaven knows where I plucked that 'you're going to be gorgeous' number from, but it was mine. Fast-forward to the day I hit the jackpot. Bingo. There was the number on the scale. But wait... nothing had changed. Sure, my jeans were slack, but I still had body hang-ups, a face covered with acne, and – the cherry on the cake – I was terrified of food.

Nowadays it's a whole new existence. I love food. I feast on delicious delights and scoff to my heart's content. I'm slimmer now than ever. Want to know the best bit? When I eat there's silence. Space. Peace. No inner nag rambling about calories, fat grams, or portion sizes. Instead my mind *oohs* and *ahs* along with me, filling me with blissful thoughts: *Oh that's so tasty and so good for you! Mmm, I love that.* There's something else, too. I did the unthinkable. I broke up with my scales: *Sorry, it's not you it's me. Well, actually, I'm lying, it's you. You make me feel bad. See ya!*

Time to jump off the crazy train

So from now on forget calories, points, fat grams, etc., because you don't need dieting jargon in your vocabulary. Scrub it and make space for better words. Let's see... how about hot, healthy, happy, and loving every minute of it? Most of us search for a superficial result. We get sucked in to believing that Botox, diets, liposuction, and fat-loss treatments will give us a killer body. We forget that the way we look is simply a mirror of our insides.

So how did I go from a diet addict/food-obsessed/bulimic/anorexic/calorie-crazed/nutcase to a health-conscious, slim, happy chick? The truth is I did one simple thing. That's it. Just one thing and it transformed my body and my relationship with food. It is by far the most powerful thing you can do if you want to have a body that rocks and a mind free from food obsession... and of course I'm going to share it with you! But wait, first I want to reveal why so many people are carrying extra junk in the trunk.

Love me a bad boy

Growing up, I loved players. If a guy seemed like the type to mess with my head, play me for a fool, and then leave me heartbroken then I wanted him bad. Charming good looks, a killer smile, and empty promises got me every time. We know these types of men are full of lies, but somehow we can't resist them. It just feels too good. We trick ourselves into believing it'll be different this time round... until we're left broken, empty. But if we had the chance, would we go back for more? Every time.

Processed foods are just like bad boys: full of promises they can't live up to. They trick our body into feeling loved, but only for an instant. They have no real depth or vital goodness. Devoid of nutrients they give a temporary feeling of pleasure that quickly vanishes, leaving us hunting down our next fix. Fancy labels, sexy packaging, and expensive advertising make us fall in love. Our biochemistry is fooled and we feel all zingy. We are hardwired to seek pleasure[1] and that is exactly what they deliver. However, they throw your blood sugar levels out of whack,[2] and that's bad news for your metabolism and your booty. We feel comforted, uplifted, and even a little numb, but only for a spell. Soon we're nose diving on the blood sugar rollercoaster, and before we know it we're lying jelly legs on the ground and scrambling for our next hit to pull us up again. We're choosing instant pleasure over long-term happiness. What was it my mother always said? You can't change them, you can only change yourself.

Fat and starving

Nowadays we're overfed and undernourished. Even homeless people are becoming obese.[3] Our foods are calorie rich and nutrient void; it's called the hunger–obesity paradox.[4] FYI, it's impossible to be hot, healthy, happy eating processed foods because you won't get specific key nutrients. Sure, processed foods taste great, but eaten in excess they can raise the risk of cancer, diabetes, heart disease, inflammation, and metabolic syndrome.[5-7] Wheat and sugar – found in the majority of processed and packaged foods – are full of empty promises: they con your body into thinking it's getting what it needs but then under-deliver on goodness. This is why you can be overweight and literally starving at a cellular level. Processed foods are highly addictive, we keep on eating, eating, and yes, eating some more and the fat piles on. Our solution? Calorie-controlled diets. These are sheer torture: eating nutrient-devoid, manufactured foods, but in limited quantities, is a living hell for the body. No wonder we can't stick to most diets. If you want to fit into those skinny jeans without the torture of deprivation, dump the processed foods.

- -

☼ *Hot, Healthy, Happy: Read food labels*

If a food contains sugar, additives, artificial flavoring, preservatives, sucralose, aspartame, milk, gluten, wheat, HFCS (high fructose corn syrup), sodium nitrate, and MSG (monosodium glutamate) then it won't give you hot, healthy, happy insides. So leave it outside and on the shelf.

- -

How to spot trouble

So perhaps it's time to say goodbye to the heartache and fall in love with real, whole foods. Natural foods are like good men. Their match.com ad would read something like this: Good old-fashioned values, vibrant and wholesome. Straightforward, kind, and versatile. Looking for someone to nourish and protect long term. Forget flying high and crashing in a hot mess. Whole foods give you long-lasting contentment. You feel nourished, cared for, and free from the agonizing mental chatter of obsession. You have energy and mental space for more. So eat for nourishment, not stimulation.

- -

☀ Hot, Healthy, Happy: Seek out the good guys

You need to be aware of the processed foods that dress up as healthy whole foods. Players faking nice guys. To avoid turmoil, get clued up on how to spot the smooth talkers from the real deal. Good, honest foods are organic, unprocessed, and unrefined. They rarely contain added ingredients, such as sugar, salt, or bad fats (see panel 'Sneaky Saboteurs' on page 24). Think about how foods used to be, created by nature before we messed with them. Consider most foods in jars, packets, boxes, or bottles as processed. Stay eagle-eyed. These do not belong in our beautiful bodies. Don't be misled by labels such as 'healthy,' 'low fat,' 'wholegrain,' 'vegetarian.' Use your head, wise one. You don't see the carrots shouting their healthy promises. Always consider what's actually in the food. Forget what the food manufacturers tell you are healthy foods. If you can't understand the ingredients, don't eat it. The end. Leave the chemistry experiments on the shelf.

- -

So does this mean you're destined to be forever cooking and preparing food from scratch? No busy lady. Fortunately there are some superstar food companies trailblazing into our lives. It tends to be the big multinationals *(you know who I'm talking about)* that serve us up the unhealthy junk. So give a standing ovation to the new wave of pioneers that have battled their way to our grocery stores and are dishing up some incredibly healthy, whole-food goodness in the shape of tasty meals and treats. A strawberry and banana smoothie is just that. No label decoding required. No e-numbers, artificial sweeteners, fillers or nasty fats included. No smoke and mirrors, no hidden agendas, just good, honest food. Some of the popular food stores have also wised up and are stocking their shelves with organic, pesticide-free goodies in safe packaging. So take notice. Take time to be informed about your grocery store's ethical policies for sourcing food (e.g. do they use free-range eggs in their pre-prepared meals, source from local suppliers, use genetically modified crops?) Read the labels and find the companies you can trust.

☼ Sneaky saboteurs

Along with being devoid of nutrients, processed foods are full of dirty little secrets in the form of additives, preservatives, and flavorings. These nasty chemicals are hiding out in many of the world's best-loved foods. Here's my worst offenders list:

Artificial sweeteners

Artificial sweeteners are safe; they don't make you fat or increase your risk of terrifying conditions... *cue evil, murderous laugh: mwah ha ha ha.* An early study linking aspartame to cancer[8] sparked a public outcry, but more recent researchers slammed it, finding artificial sweeteners to be of no risk.[9] *Shhh... sweeteners are big business, didn't you know.* But what about the fact that methanol in aspartame converts to formaldehyde? You've heard of formaldehyde, right? The stuff found in paint remover! The end product of formaldehyde is formate and an accumulation of that can cause methanol poisoning (blindness, fatal kidney damage, multiple-organ failure, and death).[10] *Not so hot for our health.* Oh, and another thing: diet soda was approved in 1983 and millions of gallons of the stuff was guzzled down, and less than a year later, brain cancer statistics skyrocketed.[11] Coincidence? The truth is that it's just too early to know the risks.

High fructose corn syrup (HFCS)

You'll find this sweetener is many foods packaged in packets, jars, or bottles. Don't be fooled. I know corn syrup sounds harmless, but it's a trap. HFCS is as addictive as white sugar, but even worse for our health. The corn used is mostly sourced from genetically modified crops – and the jury is out on those, too.

Monosodium glutamate (MSG)

Did you know MSG is actually what scientists use to fatten up mice for their experiments? Go ahead and Google MSG fat-induced mice and find out for yourself. Hardly surprisingly, it can make us fat, too.[12, 13] MSG is believed to turn off the brain receptors that tell the body it's full.[14] The gut secretes the hormone leptin to signal it's full, but even when it's screaming, the brain can no longer interpret what it's saying. Without this 'stop-eating' trigger, forget that lovely feeling of fullness after you've eaten. You're now a bottomless pit. MSG also tricks the brain into loving the taste of foods by spiking dopamine levels, which give feelings of euphoria. *How lethal is that to your waistline!* A substance that makes food taste awesome hooks your body into wanting more, and stops the mechanism that tells you to stop eating. *Mmm... yum, not!*

Side effects include headaches, dizziness, itchy skin, breathing problems, digestive, circulatory, and coronary effects.[15] You may be eating MSG at least three times a day because it is a typical ingredient in soups, sauces, desserts, skimmed and semi-skimmed milk, chewing gum, processed foods, and non-organic fruits and vegetables as a wax or pesticide. It's even in some baby milk formulas! It's hidden under at least 40 different names, making it nearly impossible for most people to identify.[16]

Partially hydrogenated vegetable oil

Heart-healthy spreads, biscuits (cookies), cakes, and crisps (chips) are made with sunflower oil, which is healthy. Or is it? Can you say trans fats for me? If you've been sucked into the margarine trap, or you love the odd cake or cookie, then the words 'partially hydrogenated

continued on p.26

continued from p.25

vegetable oil' might be important to you. This wonky, doomful mixture is concocted from vegetable oil and hydrogen, turning it into treacherous trans fats which are linked to cancer[17] and an increased risk of coronary events. Does that mean those heart-healthy spreads are actually damaging our hearts?[18] Something to ponder...

Pesticides

Almost all non-organic foods contain pesticides. In fact more than two billion pounds of pesticides are added to our food supply every year. Here's the thing: most are carcinogenic and have been linked to a number of serious health conditions including neurological, leukemia, nervous system, and reproductive disturbances.[19] *Go organic! Rah, rah!*

Sodium nitrate and nitrates

Bacon, salami, processed meat, and smoked salmon should be avoided at all costs. Laced with preservatives known as sodium nitrate and nitrates, which turn into nitrosamines, all these foods have been linked with cancer.[20]

Big fat con

In my dieting days I was terrified of fat. After all, fat makes you fat, right? Well, not exactly. Humans love to have an enemy, and as the obesity epidemic soared, so fat became the villain. We waged a war against fat. No one was safe. There was widespread panic. FAT IS MAKING US FAT! *Cue gasping sounds.* Well hello booming low-fat diet industry. Thank heavens you've swooped in to save our waistlines. Their superhero slogan: 'Want to be thin? Go low fat!' Next minute we're shaking our heads in disgust at the avocados, naughty nuts, and oils: *Tut tut. How could you do this to us?* As we lovingly ushered the plastic, fake, low-fat, sugar-laden, and artificially sweetened products into our shopping baskets in the belief they'd make us thin. But think about it: does eating fat make you fat? Of course, anything in excess does, but fat isn't the bad guy. In fact, statistics show that as our fat intake has dropped so our waistlines have grown.[21] *Huh? Something smells fishy*. If fat isn't making us fat then what foodstuff has increased in correlation to our size? You've guessed it... sugar!

☼ *Hot, Healthy, Happy: Dump diet foods*

Dump the low-fat, artificially sweetened, manufactured foods and enjoy moderate amounts of delicious, nutrient-packed raw plant fats such as avocados, cold-pressed oils, nuts, nut butters, and seeds. These foods naturally satisfy your hunger, meaning it's difficult to overeat them.

You're sweet enough

Before we dive in to how sugar is keeping you away from those skinny jeans, let's redefine it because I'm not just demonizing the white cane stuff here. I'm also talking about white breads, pasta, rice, waffles, muffins, and cereals, which all turn into glucose (aka sugar). A spoonful of sugar or a slice of bread, it's six of one and half a dozen of the other. Too much and you get excess glucose. *Psst... excess glucose makes you fat*. Here comes the science...

The human body is built for feast and famine. Who are we kidding? Famine never comes. Mother Nature didn't bargain on bakeries packed with donuts, cream cakes, and baguettes. She feared we might starve, so extra glucose is never wasted; its nicely stored as fat for a rainy day. Nowadays those rainy days never arrive and we're all getting fatter. When glucose swims in the bloodstream, the pancreas releases insulin, our fat-producing hormone. This little hormone wears many hats, but his main job is to shunt glucose into the cells for energy. But what if we're stuffing our face while trawling Facebook at our desks? If we don't use up the glucose immediately (by exercise), a danger signal is released (because too much sugar in the blood causes damage to the body's soft tissues) and the body quickly moves to plan B to prevent damage. The result? The pancreas releases insulin, which gets busy storing the glucose as fat.

A diet high in simple sugars and refined carbohydrates dumps a stack of glucose into the bloodstream. The poor pancreas goes into overdrive, shoving out more insulin. This is a dangerous cycle because eventually the exhausted cells get fed up and stop responding, leaving insulin swimming around the blood for long periods. *News flash: Your body can't lose weight with insulin streaming through your system.* When your body finally starts sucking up the glucose, your blood sugar levels plummet. Cue the headaches, irritability and anxiety, and that little voice in your head saying: *Is it snack time already?*

So what's your typical day? In fact, what's most people's typical day? Do you perhaps start with a bowl of cereal or a slice or two of wheat toast for breakfast? Mid-morning signals time for a little pick-me-up such as a cup of tea or coffee, a soda, or a chocolate bar. Is it a sandwich or pasta salad for lunch? Feeling low by mid-afternoon? Time for another pick-me-up: a piece or cake, a few cookies or white crackers? And what's for dinner... another bowl of pasta, a pizza, or some French fries or white rice with the meal? Not forgetting that sugary dessert or glass or two of sweet or medium white wine in the evening. Did you know that this type of diet has your insulin levels high for around 18 hours a day? Since insulin is your fat-producing hormone, just imagine what's happening in your body. Insulin is making fat in your cells 18 hours a day. That doesn't leave much time for breaking it down. Do you really want to be cruising in a fat-making machine?

Meet glucagon. She's your fat burner – *I'm sure she probably has a fan club you can join.* Now insulin and glucagon work different shifts. So when insulin is out running wild in the bloodstream, shy, retiring glucagon keeps her head down and has a break. You want to be slim and slender? Stop allowing insulin to run the show. Let glucagon take center stage.

Balancing your blood sugar levels throughout the day will send insulin home and glucagon can start streamlining those thighs. This is why low fat is nonsense. Imagine a wheelbarrow full of white sugar. I could whack a label on it stating '100 percent fat free.' This would be factually correct, as it has zero fat. But wait a minute: doesn't your body turn sugar directly into fat? So yes, the label is factually correct – *thank you Mr. Advertising Standards Agency* – but it means zilch to your body! An understanding of simple biochemistry and now you're free from the low-fat diet trap. I told you science was sexy.

Hot, Healthy, Happy: Balance your blood sugar

Apart from the negative effects on your waistline, high sugar intake and poor blood sugar balance have also been linked to a decline in mental ability,[22] an increase in depression, and even violence.[23, 24] So okay, the thought of giving up your beloved treats may have you breaking into a cold sweat, but here's the upside. You could be left happier (yes, really), slimmer, more chilled, and (dare I say) a little smarter. The good news is that you can still eat 'treats' on the HHH 21-day diet, but you might need to give your snack cupboard a makeover first. When you do, you'll soon see the benefits because when your blood sugar is stellar you'll feel satisfied. Hunger is genuine hunger. No more blood sugar crashes, running to the local store for a fix of chocolate, or stalking the vending machine from the post-lunch zonked zone.

Want to get skinny and sexy? Stop living on stimulation. Full stop. No excuses. Dump the nicotine, alcohol, and stress. Get organized and slow down. Yes, being late will make you fat! And we'll be talking more about that in the next chapter when you'll be learning how to eat yourself happy.

My secret weapon for carb lovers

So before you think I'm going all Atkins on you, let's get you up to speed. Do not fear, carb maniacs, there is a way to eat carbs and stay trim. Carbohydrates are usually labeled under complex (gorgeously good or unrefined) and simple (bad, useless, or refined). Complex carbs are your whole grains, beans, legumes, and veggies. They take longer to digest so your blood sugar levels stay steady, meaning no more blood sugar rollercoasters and, not surprisingly, they're better for weight loss. They're also packed with lots of good stuff such as vitamins, minerals, enzymes, protein, and fiber. The first step is switching to whole varieties, but remember you'll still need to watch the quantities because all carbs turn to sugar if they're not used up running to the health food store.

To navigate the carbs world I'd like to introduce you to my secret weapon – 'glycemic load' (GL). The GL is a relatively new way to determine the impact carbs have on the body. In the past glycemic index (GI) was all the rage. Unfortunately that only tells you how rapidly a carbohydrate will turn into sugar – it doesn't account for the amount of carbohydrate in the food. For example, let's take a big delicious juicy slice of watermelon. The carbohydrate in the watermelon turns quickly to glucose in the body, giving it a high GI, so following the GI concept, you would pass on the watermelon. However, a watermelon has very little carbohydrate so it doesn't do much to your blood sugar levels. Great news... I love watermelons!

The truth is we need to know both: how fast releasing the carbohydrate is and how much carbohydrate there is in it. You need both pieces of the puzzle to understand its effect, which is why low GL rocks. In fact, low-GL diets have been found to decrease the risk of diabetes,[25–27] cancer,[28] and have a dazzling effect on your midriff.[29-30] Low-GL foods are also better at curbing appetite compared to low-calorie and low-fat diets.[31] The HHH 21-day diet is packed with low-GL goodies, ideal for keeping that blood sugar balanced and smiling.

☼ *Hot, Healthy, Happy: Eat low-GL carbs*

Escape the blood sugar rollercoaster by eating low-GL carbohydrates (whole grains, beans, legumes, pulses, and veggies), raw plant fats, and good quality proteins every three to four hours. Dump the stimulants, stress, and sugar. Depending on how you eat at the moment, this could seem like a big change. That's okay. Give yourself time. The HHH 21-day diet will naturally help you to overcome cravings for those sugar-laden carbs and give you more energy so you won't need the stimulants. Over time, choosing the HHH foods will become second nature, as your body will intuitively seek out foods that don't spike your sugar levels and leave you feeling satisfied and calm. For now, just lean into it.

Be a gluten-free goddess

If you feel lousy no matter what, it's likely that gluten is your enemy. Gluten is a protein found in wheat, barley, spelt, kamut, and rye, and many people are gluten intolerant. However, it's estimated that 99 percent of people who have a problem with eating it, don't even know it.[32] Not only can it destroy your waistline, gluten intolerance is also associated with osteoporosis, irritable bowel syndrome (IBS), cancer,[33] depression, anxiety,[34] dementia,[35] and migraines.[36] One review linked gluten with over 55 diseases![37] Hidden gluten sensitivity can even increase your risk of death by 35–75 percent, mostly by causing heart disease and cancer.[38] I'll reveal more about divine digestion in Chapter 3 (see pages 59–60), but cutting out gluten can be one of the most powerful things you can do if you have digestive issues.

So maybe it's time to wave farewell. Breakups can be tough, I hear you. It's true, the pasta, cereal, bread, and almost all the processed foods will need to go, but your body and your skinny jeans will thank you for it.

☀ *Hot, Healthy, Happy: Get a new brand*

If you think life without gluten just isn't worth living then I've got good news – just switch your brand. There are loads of lovely gluten-free products available, just don't get caught in the gluten-free junk food trap (gluten-free cakes, macaroons, and cookies are still cakes, macaroons, and cookies). Instead, discover natural gluten-free grains such as quinoa, buckwheat, millet, amaranth, brown and wild rice. You can even buy brown rice pasta, buckwheat, and quinoa breads. Oats can sometimes be contaminated so opt for gluten-free varieties. There are also loads of delicious gluten-free granolas to choose from, and for baking opt for gluten-free flours. Remember, fruits, greens, veggies, beans, pulses, sweet potatoes, seeds, and nuts don't have a smidgen of gluten, so fill up on these health-giving stars of the show.

Going against the grain

Wheat is the Louis Vuitton of foods: 'I love bread, I dream about it.' You're hooked on it, right? We're told that wheat is a natural, fiber-rich food. *Blah, blah, blah.* But the wheat dressed up as fancy foods lining the grocery store's shelves is far from the wheat your great granny would have used.[39] Oh no, you're eating the Frankenstein of wheat. The problem is that most manufacturers opt for looks over integrity when it comes to wheat and cereal products; they figured out some time ago that we preferred their products when they were white and soft, and so they strip the natural grains to within an inch of their lives. Goodbye nutrients, vitamins, minerals, natural goodness, sparkle, and life force. The worldwide food standards agencies recognized the consequences and now manufacturers have to 'enrich' and 'fortify' their products. But Mother Nature isn't an idiot and our bodies can't absorb these minerals as easily[24]. This chemically engineered, unnatural monster causes a cascade of chronic illnesses. It's time to liberate and I can think of three reasons why you absolutely should.

1. Genetic alteration and hybridization mean that wheat is now richer in a starch called amylopectin A.[39] Sure, it looks appetizing, but a slice of whole grain bread or a bowl of cereal spikes your blood sugar levels by more than a tablespoon of sugar. So you see Mr. Cereal Giant, slapping a healthy 'whole grain' label on a processed food, high in sugar and refined wheat, is just rubbish.

2. Commercially produced wheat is packed with double the number of chromosomes of a large variety of gluten proteins, which have soared from 4 to 14 percent over the last 100 years.[40] Gluten is one of the worst offenders for damaging the gut lining[41] as it increases zonulin, which has been found to create leaky gut.[42] Leaky gut has been linked to bowel disease,[43-49] acne, and psoriasis,[50] and many more health issues. So if you ever wondered why you feel bloated and uncomfortable after eating that sandwich or bowl of cereal, now you know why.

3. Gluten also has a drug-like effect on the body and drives us crazy with cravings, so it's the ultimate bad boy for keeping us hooked and hungry for more. When it hits the gut, the proteins shorten into polypeptides, aka exorphin[51], or morphine-like compounds. That's right, they literally turn you into a crackhead. Binding to opioid receptors in the brain, they hook you like a drug addict. The dominant ones,

which cross your blood–brain barrier, are gluteomorphins, named after 'gluten' and 'morphine.' So not only does it have you bingeing on toasties and face-planting donuts, it can increase your risk of mental health problems, too.

- -

☀ *Hot, Healthy, Happy: Give gluten-free living a go*

Go on: give it a whirl, just for 21 days. Don't make me beg, it isn't ladylike. Think of it as an adventure. Head to your local grocery/ health food store and discover all the wonderful substitutes that are gluten free: pasta, pizza bases, breads, cereals, and more. Pick whatever tickles your fancy and then simply make the switch. Notice how your digestive system, skin, moods, and sleep are transformed. And if that isn't incentive enough, cutting gluten out of your diet means you'll lose that bloated feeling within a week – *hello, naturally flat tummy, where have you been hiding...*

- -

Think yourself skinny

Still wondering about that one simple thing I did that transformed my weight? Here it is... I changed my focus. That's it. Simply shift your focus away from dieting and give some time and effort to why you're out of balance. To end obsession you need to know who you are. You need to discover what powers you up and what crashes your system.

Many years ago I stopped thinking about dieting and started to consider why my body was overweight, unhappy, and stressed out. I began to listen to what it had to say. I noticed that so many parts of my body and life were off kilter. Processed foods, artificial sweeteners, sugar-loving yeasts, food cravings, toxic build up, nutrient deficiencies, negative thinking, poor boundaries, gut rumbles, and hormonal havoc. These were why I was fat, sick, and tired. Not lack of willpower or the wrong diet plan!

☀ *Hot, Healthy, Happy: Overwhelm is not part of the plan*

All the information in this chapter is designed to empower you, not overwhelm you. We all have busy lives, and eating well and staying healthy enables us to have the energy and stamina to follow our dreams. So if you feel stressed out by the thought of the work you need to do to get the body you want, stop. Take a breath. Simply focus on what small changes you could make today that would change how you feel and look tomorrow. The road to success is paved with small, daily actions. Make this your starting goal to shift your focus to health.

A healthy body is naturally skinny. Shoot for health and the pounds will fall away. That's what the HHH 21-day diet is all about: it is a journey of self-discovery to help you identify the imbalances keeping you stuck. If you're living with excess pounds, they'll shift. The key is to stop thinking about the weight. Focus on getting healthy, happy, and most importantly, hot! Let that be your North Star.

Hot, Healthy, Happy action plan

- ♥ Change your focus to getting healthy, not just losing weight.

- ♥ Start dumping processed foods with their sneaky chemicals. It's time to fall in love with real, whole foods.

- ♥ Remember that nutrient deficiencies create cravings. Ask yourself whenever you eat something: is this food packed with micronutrients? Am I filling myself up with nourishment or stimulation?

- Start noticing what stimulants you use to keep you going. Swap your coffee or black tea for herbal teas, and soft drinks for fresh juices or just water with a squeeze of orange or lemon juice.

- Since fat doesn't make you fat, how about dumping the low-fat products and filling up with good quality fats – delicious avocados, nuts, and seeds?

- Are you ready to escape the blood sugar rollercoaster? Then dump the nutrient-devoid refined white carbs and replace them with low glycemic load (GL) carbohydrates, e.g. fresh, green leafy vegetables, fruits (berries, apples, pears), and complex carbohydrates, e.g. quinoa, buckwheat, millet, brown basmati rice, sweet potatoes, beans, and pulses.

- Aim to eat every three to fours hours to keep your brain nourished and maintain your energy levels.

- Finally say goodbye to gluten (wheat, barley, rye, and spelt) and become a gluten-free goddess.

Chapter 2

Eat Yourself Happy: Turning Dark Moods Technicolor

Fed up with feeling out of control around food? Depressed, anxious, guilty, or irritated about your life? Before you hit eBay in search of a personality transplant, know that hope is not lost because I was there, too. Confidence, happiness, motivation, determination, and contentment aren't just personality traits with which a lucky few are born. You can possess any or even all of these. Want to liberate your hidden talents? But first, another admission:

Worrier. Obsessive. Perfectionistic. These were my defining characteristics. My secret talent: the ability to take something totally insignificant and worry about it... endlessly. My best friends were anxiety and panic. *You may have met them.* Guilt lived next door: the unwelcome guest who would pop over whenever I was enjoying myself a little too much. Obsession followed me around like a shadow. Some people are obsessively tidy and organized. *Ha! If only.* No tidy rooms for me, I was too busy managing body obsessions and mirror issues. In fact, I worried about not being obsessed about being tidy. *Go figure.* Terrorizing myself was an everyday pastime. At night my neurotic mind kept me from peaceful sleep. I was Little Miss High Achiever, but in reality no accomplishment satisfied me. The worst of it was that I was ruled by food cravings. Dieting all day then haunted by food demons reciting the contents of my refrigerator all night: images of leftovers hijacking my good intentions. Of course I thought everyone else was fine, it was just me. But I feared the worst... I thought I might be nuts.

Today I'm a chilled chick (well, mostly!). I discovered there was more to it than a personality fault. My biochemistry was out of sorts and in desperate need of a reboot. I also know now that I wasn't the only one. Many of us ride the negative rollercoaster of stress, worry, and mood swings. Every day in my clinic room I meet clients who spend their days feeling the way I once did. Overwhelmed by their responsibilities and underwhelmed by their life. They feel anxious for no reason: living in a stress response and struggling to switch off. It is fabulous to see them transform, chill out, and start to enjoy their lives more as they change their diet and lifestyle. Now it's your turn.

Dark moods and food cravings can simply be an imbalance in brain chemicals, and this chapter will explain the three main imbalances – which many people suffer from, not just you or me in my distant past – and how to remedy them using the HHH 21-day diet. You don't need willpower or Prozac, just give your brain what she's really missing: give your plate a makeover, curb cravings, and charge your brain for happiness, confidence, pleasure, and contentment. Let's shake away cravings, ramp up your feel-good chemicals, and turn those dark moods technicolor. But first you might find it helpful to know a little more about how your brain chemistry works.

You versus your brain

Your brain is a hive of disco-dancing electric activity. Right now more than 100,000 chemical reactions are getting groovy.

What you think, feel, and do is determined by your brain's communication skills with your nerve cells. Its messengers are called neurotransmitters (aka your feel-good chemicals). Whether you feel alert, happy, motivated, calm, stressed, or irritated depends on which messengers are on duty. You choose your mood with your food because what you eat determines which messengers run the show. Before we dig into how these affect your appetite, mood, and even cravings, let's get up to speed with how your brain works its magic.

Meet your brain. Beware, she's a balance freak. Overly stressed and she steers you to trigger the release of calming messengers. An angry outburst, a large cocktail, watching soaps, dancing, maybe face-planting a chocolate cake, what's your brain's stress-relieving recipe? She's also a pleasure seeker (dare I say pleasure addict). That desirable willpower you're after is a scrawny contender alongside your brain's butched-up desire for pleasure and balance. During emotional torment or stress she'll literally nag you for instant relief. A fast learner who prefers tried-and-tested methods: that donut brought oozing pleasure last time so eat one now! The smell, look, taste, and texture of food can all excite our brain chemicals for pleasure, calm, and emotional deliciousness. If it gives you quick and instantaneous pleasure, the brain wants it again and again and again.

Sadly, the foods we crave are often the very reason why we feel self-loathing, depressed, and fat in the first place. Your brain would have you riding that merry-go-round of cravings, bingeing, pleasure, guilt day in day out, but before you can jump for freedom you need to ask yourself: 'Can you outsmart your brain?' Can you change your responses, outwit her and reprogram better choices? Once you do this you can stop looking for balance and pleasure at the bottom of the ice-cream tub.

Type 1: Living under a rain cloud

Do you sometimes feel as if you're living under a rain cloud of negativity? If depression and anxiety are round for regular sleepovers, you can suspect it's not you but rather that serotonin is in short supply. She's your happy messenger: confident, chilled, positive, smiling, happy, and sparkling. High serotonin levels mean you'll ooze superstar. Who wouldn't want a piece of that? With her there's no room for doom and gloom. Without her in your life, you might find that perfectionism has you rocking the high-achiever status while secretly suspecting a personality defect or popping serotonin-boosting pills such as Prozac. However the symptoms are manifesting, low serotonin means you'll be feeling lackluster,[1] and may be experiencing some or all of the following symptoms:

- ❤ Premenstrual syndrome (PMS)

- ❤ Panic

- ❤ Irritability

- ❤ Anxiety

- ❤ Constipation

- ❤ Worry

- ❤ Insomnia

- ❤ Depression[2]

- ❤ Muscle pain

How did you and serotonin lose touch?

If you're camped-out indoors most days then your serotonin levels are likely to be low because sunshine boosts serotonin production.[3] Particularly in the winter, when the dark nights roll in, low serotonin can have us on the sofa surfing carbs and perhaps even feeling SAD (seasonal affective disorder). Even on a sunny day you may not be getting enough light. A sunny day between April and September gives around 100,000 lux. If you spend most of your time inside or, depending on where you live, during the winter months you'll get less than 100 lux.[4] Combat this with bright lamp therapy in the shape of a good quality light box. Fantastic for SAD[5], and even for non-seasonal depression.[6,7]

A lack of pro-serotonin foods in your diet, such as protein and essential fatty acids, low-calorie diets and skipping meals can also dwindle your levels. Other serotonin saboteurs are stress, caffeinated drinks, diet drinks or foods. Finally, your sex hormones may be out of sorts, but I'll be showing you the way to hormone harmony in the next chapter.

☼ Hot, Healthy, Happy: Naturally boost your day

Cutting out stimulants and processed foods is vital for beating the blues. Stress also depletes your serotonin reserves, as your brain struggles to meet the overwhelming daily demands, so consider a daily practice such as meditation to help you feel calmer throughout the day. You might like to start by using my simple guide to meditation in Part IV (see pages 169–170).

Boost serotonin production by shining some more light into your life: aim to spend at least 20 minutes outside in the fresh air every day. In the winter months, or if you live in a cooler climate where the sun rarely shines, invest in a good quality light box. Soak up the light for 30–60 minutes every day and enjoy the blissful sensation of serotonin running riot in your brain.

Understanding low serotonin

Want to feel more positive, happy, and content? Then have a serotonin recharge. When serotonin drops, your brain doesn't have a magical 'aha' moment and reach for the protein and essential fats. It's a pleasure addict. Forget long-term gratification, it wants the quick hit NOW – the instant boost to *Ahhh*. Say hello carbohydrate cravings. Serotonin is one of the reasons why carbs are so comforting – because they give us a serotonin high.[8, 9] Just been dumped? Bad haircut? Had a row with a friend? Cake is the ultimate therapy.

☀ Beware the vicious cycle

Here's how serotonin works: think rugby players (small shorts and all). Tryptophan is the wee geeky guy at the back trying to get through to the try line. When tryptophan tries to compete with all the other amino acids to get through your blood–brain barrier, he gets pushed out the way. When you dose yourself up on sugars and refined carbohydrates (e.g. a bowl of milky cereal or buttery wheat toast), your pancreas spurts out insulin, your blood sugar levels spike and insulin shunts the other amino acids out of your bloodstream, giving tryptophan the whole playing field to himself. No more being shoved to the back, he now gets a free ride straight to your brain. He converts to 5-HTP, then to serotonin.[10] In response we scoff sugary carbs and get a hit of pleasure. However, as discussed in the previous chapter, spiked blood sugar means excess glucose and the inevitable stored pounds (see pages 27–28). Your blood sugar levels plummet and you're back feeling depressed, stressed, and anxious. Where did those cakes go again? It's time to jump off that merry-go-round, honey. Serotonin levels drop as a result of poor diet, lack of sunshine, overdoing the anti-serotonin foods, imbalanced sex hormones, and stress overload. The result? More cravings for carbohydrates and fats to regain that calm feeling again.

Are you a serotonin junkie?
Low moods, yo-yo dieting, excess weight, and carb fests can have us spinning in a Bermuda Triangle-type vortex of doom; they're all

inter-linked.[11,12] Overwhelmed and undernourished, we feel low so the brain tells us to use carbohydrates as an emotional pick-me-up. Before we know it, we're back in our fat jeans. Are you ready to check your brain into food rehab? Outsmart her? What if you didn't wait until the body was low in serotonin and your brain was crying out for cream cakes? What if every day you chose to consistently nourish your body with pro-serotonin foods to balance your blood sugar levels, nourish it with vitamins, minerals, protein, and essential fats? What would life be like without the constant cravings, out-of-control feelings, pessimism, and negativity? What could you achieve once you were no longer caught in the depressed, binge, guilt trap? Imagine if you were a high serotonin superstar: glowing, positive, chilled out, smiling, and happy.

- -

☼ *Hot, Healthy, Happy: Eat more serotonin-boosting foods*

Get out from under the rain cloud by getting your body to make its very own happy. Serotonin is made from the amino acid (protein building block) tryptophan. You'll find tryptophan in the following foods: brown rice, nuts, avocados, eggs, almonds, oily fish, fruit, and green leafy vegetables.

The HHH 21-day diet is packed with these happy foods. Once in your body they're turned into 5-HTP, which converts to serotonin.[13] *Hey presto, happy lady.* For an instant fix you could also take 50mg of 5-HTP daily: take 1–3 supplements mid-afternoon and 1–3 again before bedtime. Your body makes 5-HTP, but only if it has enough tryptophan. 5-HTP increases your levels of serotonin[14] and has been found to help with the blues[15] even more than SSRIs.

CAUTION: *5-HTP is not suitable for people on certain medications such as anti-depressants. Always check with your medical practitioner before introducing supplements.*

- -

Type 2: Sleeping your way through life

It's 7 a.m., the alarm is screeching. Most mornings we should jump out of bed and skip out the door singing isn't life awesome? However, if it's more like groan, stumble downstairs, and throw back a coffee before opening your eyes you could have lost your energizing messengers. Other symptoms might be:

- Life feels a drag – dull, uninteresting, and boring.
- Rather than highly-strung and irritated by everyone, you feel *nada*.
- You might sit in silence around others, or feel shy and unable to come out of your shell.

If any of these sound familiar, perhaps it's not you, perhaps it's your brain and it sounds as if she's in need of a boost.

Let me explain: serotonin is your happy messenger but the catecholamines (dopamine, norephrine, and adrenalin) are your energizers.[4] These live wires give you oomph, drive, and zest. They keep you firing hot and fierce emotionally, mentally, and physically: raring to go, upbeat, focused, clear, and motivated.[13] Dopamine is the top guy responsible for producing the other two. Feeling psyched about that big date, pumped about that overseas trip, eagerly anticipating Saturday night's party? Catecholamines are your cheer squad revving you on. They also keep you alert and ready for action. A spat with a frenemy, running late for that big gig, or just heard some bad news, they keep you on edge. Therefore, being outgoing or shy can also be determined by how much of these catecholamines your brain is producing. How amazing is that! Not only can you eat yourself happy, you can also eat yourself confident. Fill up on these brain chemicals and watch your biochemistry liven up, shimmer, and steal the show.

Another telltale sign that you're low in these energizing chemicals is a love of stimulants. What's your drug of choice? Is it a hot steaming cup of Joe, a frappamochachino with a double shot of espresso, the odd joint, a cheeky cigarette, a beer or a snort of crack? What do you rely on to help you kickass? Cravings for these stimulants are just your body's way of getting an instant boost in your energizing brain chemicals.[16] Let's give your brain a natural boost. Catecholamines are made from the amino acid tyrosine[17], an awesome happy chemical. Tyrosine produces our live-wire chemicals and is the raw ingredient for our adrenal glands (aka the body's stress management center). Tyrosine is packed high in protein rich foods, and so a high-GL diet, skipping meals, or living on processed foods can result in less than optimum levels. This is because a spike in blood sugar levels shunts tyrosine out of the bloodstream.

- -

☀ *Hot, Healthy, Happy: Boost your tyrosine intake*

Want a boost without the caffeine or stimulants? The HHH 21-day diet is packed with foods rich in tyrosine (e.g. eggs, fish, green leafy vegetables, avocados, and almonds). If you still find you need more of a boost then try supplementing daily with 1000mg of tyrosine (see caution below) first thing in the morning.[16] If you feel jittery you've overdone it.

If you're still not feeling so hot then ask your medical practitioner to test your thyroid (or visit www.thefoodpsychologist.com). A sluggish thyroid means your brain won't be getting enough T3 to build your energizing chemicals. A number of studies have found tyrosine to be useful during conditions of stress, cold, fatigue,[20] loss of a loved one (e.g. in death or divorce), prolonged work, and sleep deprivation,[21, 22] as it reduces stress hormone levels.[23]

CAUTION: *Tyrosine is not suitable for people with high blood pressure. Always check with your medical practitioner before introducing supplements.*

- -

Stress can also deplete levels, while foods like soy can actually inhibit tyrosine.[18] This is bad news for vegetarians substituting a high meat diet with a high soy diet. Exercise also boosts not only serotonin[19] but catecholamine levels, too. But let's face it, if you're low in these, then it's likely that exercise is probably the last thing on your agenda!

Type 3: Acting tough or oversensitive?

Some people love life. Everything is bliss. Faced with painful stuff they come back like a boomerang. They're loaded with brain chemicals called endorphins. More powerful than morphine and heroin, these inborn bliss chemicals ramp up pleasure and make pain bearable. The tingle when you fall head over heels in love, that euphoric feeling at the mere mention of chocolate, or that 'ah' moment when you step into a hot bath, that's your endorphins talking. To find out if you're rocking low levels, answer the following questions:

- ♥ Have you lost your joy for life?

- ♥ Do you act tough to keep others away?

- ♥ Do you pretend things are great, while crumbling inside?

- ♥ Does the thought of getting close to someone terrify you?

- ♥ Would you do anything to avoid confrontation?

- ♥ Are you overly sensitive to pain or discomfort, and get upset easily?

- ♥ Do you regularly seek comfort in chocolate, alcohol, painkillers, and drugs?

If you answered yes to more than a couple of these questions, then you may be low in your pleasure chemicals. How did that happen? It is possible you were born deficient, particularly if you've always been 'the sensitive one.' Or you might have been a happy-go-lucky kid but emotional and physical pain and stress have drained your endorphins.

The good news is these reserves can be rebuilt. According to Julia Ross in *The Mood Cure*⁴, the magic formula is DLPA found in high-protein foods. Your happy chemical serotonin, and its creator 5-HTP, also stimulate your endorphins, so 5-HTP and DLPA is the ultimate combo to have you dancing on rainbows.

☼ *Hot, Healthy, Happy: Spice it up, hot stuff*

Throw some spices into your daily cuisine (e.g. cumin, coriander/cilantro, and turmeric) because these are believed to boost endorphins. The HHH 21-day diet is also packed with fresh whole foods rich in proteins, vitamins, and minerals essential for rebalancing your system. If you want an extra endorphin boost, then supplement with 1–2 DLPA 500mg (250mg D, 250mg L) in the morning, mid-morning, and mid-afternoon.

CAUTION: *DLPA may not be suitable for people with certain medical conditions or those taking medications. Always check with your medical practitioner before introducing supplements.*

Getting high on cookie dough ice cream

So give up the old ways and your brain's naughty pleasures, whether it's pizza, cheese, ice cream, or cake? Think about how you feel after eating them: bloated, gassy, sleepy, sneezy, sore throat. If they make you feel sick why do you keep eating them? We're intelligent and sophisticated, obviously, but we make bad food choices again and again. What's going on? Remember, the brain is a pleasure addict and these foods trigger our pleasure chemicals.

At 17, my tried-and-tested endorphin high was a carton of cookie dough ice cream. It had me rolling in happy land. The chocolate is packed with sugar and drug-like substances salsolinol, theobromine, caffeine, PEA, and anandamide (a marijuana-like brain chemical), wheat flour, and milk. All of these ingredients locked into my endorphin receptors and lit me up like a Christmas tree. It was the ultimate big hitter: milk, flour, sugar, and chocolate. These all create inflammation by triggering the release of false endorphins called exorphins[24, 25] which harm the body, and so the brain tries to restore balance. That's right, pleasure chemicals make bad food pleasurable, which is why dieting or eliminating foods can be so difficult. The brain misses all those feel-good chemicals and makes us crave more. So you must outsmart your brain if you want to lose weight and feel bodacious.

Conquer cravings

The truth is, some foods have drug-like effects on us. When you think milk and gluten, think LSD-style effects. Remember gluten and its gluteomorphins from the previous chapter (see pages 31–34)? Well, dairy has caseomorphins that, like gluteomorphins, have an opioid effect[26], and produces a state of euphoria. Mother Nature gave dairy opioid effects to help babies space out and doze off after feeds.[27] Cheese is super addictive because it is concentrated casein and fat, which means high levels of opiates. It also contains phenylethylamine (PEA), an amphetamine-like chemical. So cheese toasties are a gluteomorphin and caseomorphin love fest! We're actually not joking when we say we're hooked on them.

However, with such powerful effects it's hardly surprising that we use food to boost our mood. Does the mere mention of chocolate give you a rush of euphoria? How often do you find yourself self-medicating your unhappiness? Forget pills and prescriptions, I'm talking cake, chocolate, and pastries? These foods patch up emotional issues, making us feel better temporarily. How much time do you spend feeling guilty around food? You're smart, you know certain foods are not helping you look and feel like a superstar, but your cravings are in the driving seat. This isn't about willpower. You're not weak-willed or faulty. Cravings are a reflection of how well we've nourished our bodies. If you're missing nourishment, your body will try to meet that deficiency.

Our brain chemicals can change every day, influencing our cravings. Remember your brain is a balance freak, so the last thing she wants is to feel upset, stressed, or guilty. She wants the quick, instant feeling of pleasure. We're often not even aware of what's happening. We feel a little down and the next minute, we're stuffing a pastry or a chocolate bar down our throats. Of course common sense tells us unhealthy foods aren't going to solve our problems, but that's far from our mind when the brain is screaming 'eat that now, I need to calm down!' Maybe when a craving hits, your approach is to ride out the urge. How long does that last? You can't ignore these urges forever. Your brain will talk you out of it. Does the term 'yo-yo dieting' sound familiar?

Instead of deprivation and restraint, work on keeping your brain happy. Arm it with the building blocks to make its feel-good chemicals, so when life does hit a downturn your biochemistry is charged for keeping you afloat.

Hot, Healthy, Happy action plan

♥   Keep balancing those blood sugar levels. This is vital for giving you a steady supply of energy and keeping moods stable.

♥   Make sure you eat good quality protein. This doesn't need to be animal protein. Plants are full of incredible protein. My favorites are quinoa, buckwheat, millet, amaranth, spirulina, nuts, seeds, beans, and pulses.

- ♥ Avoid low-calories diets and skipping meals!

- ♥ With a high-plant diet you should be getting lots of lovely essential fatty acids from cold-pressed oils, nuts, seeds, and raw plant fats such as avocados. This can help increase the production of feel-good messengers.

- ♥ Hopefully, you've already dumped the processed foods. If not this should give you even more incentive. Eliminate pro-inflammatory and bad-mood foods and drinks (e.g. dairy, coffee, gluten, bad fats, refined white flour, alcohol, and refined sugar). Serotonin saboteurs such as caffeine, nicotine, and artificial sweeteners, in particular, deplete your body of nutrients essential for converting tryptophan to 5-HTP to serotonin. Without calcium, magnesium, vitamin D, and B vitamins you won't keep churning out the neurotransmitters.

- ♥ We'll be going into how to manage stress in Part III because your happy chemicals can become depleted with stress: it saps your serotonin, catecholamines, and endorphins.

- ♥ Balance your hormone levels if these are out of sorts because your neurotransmitters can be affected. You'll discover the secrets of hormone balance in Chapter 4.

- ♥ Finally, it's time to start shaking that booty. During exercise, amino acids are shunted into your muscles for muscle repair, leaving tryptophan to get a free ride to the brain where it converts to 5-HTP then serotonin: runners' high, laughing after Zumba, or skipping out of the gym are all thanks to increased serotonin. If you are addicted to exercise you might want to give DLPA a go and pull your exercise plan back to more moderate levels, more on that in Chapter 4.

Chapter 3

Do You Have the Guts to be Healthy?

How often do you sit on the throne? Once a week? Every other day? Did you know that we're meant to 'go' to the bathroom two or three times a day? In an ideal world, natural whole foods go in, the body takes what it needs to make us delicious and the rest is eliminated without a fuss. For each meal we should go to the toilet. If you don't, you're not alone because it seems almost everyone nowadays is constipated. What about swelling up like a pregnant chick after only a mouthful of food? Cramping when it's not even your time of the month? Or secretly suffering with flatulence?

If you're slugging around waste in your cells, tissues, and colon you're destroying your radiant potential. Junk foods bung up your system, mess with your immune system, and turn the body into a human petri dish of pathogens. It's not a good thought, but if your internal plumbing is faulty, then your health will suffer, you'll be hauling around extra pounds, and your skin won't glow. To be hot, healthy, happy you have to have divine digestion, so this chapter is about how to temper the road rage on our internal highway. I'm also going to reveal an incredible four-step formula that is the golden ticket to divine digestion. Warning: we're going to talk excrement. Let's get down and dirty. Your vitality and glow depend on it.

Food quarantine

Let's begin with a magical guided tour. Your fabulous digestive system is employed by your body to extract nutrients from your food and package the leftover waste for elimination. This process starts at your mouth and finishes with a little package in your toilet pan. *Ooh la la.* The whole adventure is a rollercoaster ride of biochemical excitement. As that yummy food enters your mouth, chewing produces enzymes in the saliva, which begins breaking down the food. This is why eating on the run is not so hot, because often we forget to chew!

After being swallowed, the food spirals down the esophagus into your stomach. This is where the real fun begins. The stomach is food quarantine. Its job is to destroy bacteria and pathogen invaders smuggling themselves into your system on your food. The stomach wages war on these nasties by hosing them down with hydrochloric acid. The pancreas is called for back up and its digestive enzymes and bicarbonate give the digestive process extra oomph later on down the line. This also breaks up the food so the gut can suck up those lovely nutrients.

Your stomach acid is the officer in charge of the body's passport control. It dictates what enters and leaves. The first passport office is situated at the entry point to your stomach – the lower esophageal sphincter (LES) valve. In a perfect scenario, as the quarantine system kicks into action, the acid shouts out to the LES valve to close over. However, if your acid levels are too weak, the valve doesn't respond. An open valve means acid can splash up toward the throat. *Hello acid reflux, heartburn, and indigestion.* The second passport control office is located between the stomach and intestines – the pyloric sphincter. If the quarantine system is on the blink, acid levels are too low to kill the invaders and passport control is barricaded. Ever wondered why you get that heavy feeling after eating, as if food is just lying about in your stomach? Sorry, passport control is closed this evening.

- -

☼ *Hot, Healthy, Happy: Fire up your food quarantine*

Start by introducing fermented foods such as cultured vegetables and apple cider vinegar to meals. Sipping apple cider vinegar mixed with a little water can really aid digestion. You can also supplement the digestive juices by taking betaine, pepsin, and digestive enzymes. Look for supplements that combine a range of plant enzymes. You will find some that also contain pepsin and hydrochloric acid (HCL) for extra oomph. Check out www.thefoodpsychologist.com for the ones I recommend.

CAUTION: *HCL, pepsin, and digestive enzymes are not suitable for those suffering with gastritis or ulcers, or on certain medications. Always check with your medical practitioner before introducing supplements.*

- -

Your wellness juju

Stomach acid is your wellness *juju*. It's vital for health. If your body can't produce enough stomach acid things go belly up. Your quarantine system goes on the fritz and nasty pathogens run 'gung ho' into your intestines and set up camps. In fact if your stomach's PH isn't lower than 2.5 then it won't kill the villains such as helicobacter or E-coli.[1] That's not all; stomach acid is also vital for breaking down your food. Without it you can become protein malnourished and can't absorb vital vitamins and minerals.[2–4] If you want gorgeous skin, hair, and nails you absolutely need plenty of delicious minerals and good quality protein, so stomach acid is crucial.

Badly digested protein is also bad news for the digestive system as it turns it into a toxic sewer. As a result blood becomes acidic since protein is acidic. How does the body deal with acidic blood? It strives to neutralize it of course. This isn't great news for our bones, however, because it has to rob them of alkalizing minerals, some of the very nutrients we need to make stomach acid in the first place. Soon you are swept into a swirling intergalactic black hole of low stomach acid: low hydrochloric acid = low minerals = acidic blood = low minerals = low stomach acid.

⚡ Acid reflux, heartburn, and indigestion

If you suffer from acid reflux it could be that your stomach acid levels are too low. Using antacids, proton pump inhibitors, and H2-receptor antagonists may ease the immediate discomfort but at what cost? Low stomach acid equals digestive disease. Don't be palmed off with a prescription of acid blockers just to 'see if it helps.' It's more important to discover the root cause of symptoms. Always rule out helicobacter pylori, hiatus hernia, and food intolerances. Moreover, research has found that a supplement containing melatonin, l-tryptophan, vitamin B6, folic acid, vitamin B12, methionine, and betaine was superior to omeprazole (an acid blocker) in the treatment of gastroesophageal reflux disease,[5] so adjusting your diet could be key in overcoming the issue.

Downward spiral

If you're caught in the dangerous circle of low stomach acid, there is an avalanche of consequences. First you could be living on steak and still be protein malnourished. The body deals with this by shooting up your cortisol levels (which is not ideal because cortisol is the grim reaper death hormone). High cortisol throws us onto a blood sugar rollercoaster and straps us in tight. *Well hello, Miss Irritability, feeling strung out? Then throw me some donuts, I'm about to crash.* Over time, your adrenal glands get fried. If you haven't heard of your adrenals before just think of them as your body's CEO of stress management. They're in charge of how you cope with stress, or don't as the case may be. Overworking your adrenals with insufficient rest, too much stress, and overdoing stimulants means risking burn out (e.g. adrenal fatigue). Apart from feeling tired and wired, the youth hormone DHEA also plummets,[6] and no one wants to look old before their time.

So you see it's vital for our food quarantine to be running smoothly. Despite the myriad of health problems low stomach acid can cause, most medics rarely take it seriously and, as a result, it's often misdiagnosed: it produces similar symptoms to gastric ulcers and hyperacidity. However, with low stomach acid, expect symptoms straight after your meal. If it's an overproduction of acid you are more likely to feel it one to six hours after eating, or during the night.

⚡ Do you have low stomach acid?

Here are some common symptoms:

* Bloating, burping, and flatulence after meals
* Heartburn, indigestion, or acid reflux
* Undigested food in stools
* Constipation or diarrhea
* Itchy anus
* Acne
* Yeast infections
* Food intolerances
* Adrenal or chronic fatigue
* Iron deficiency
* Hair loss
* Dry skin
* Autoimmune conditions

Still not sure, then take the test!

Make sure your tummy is empty. Add a teaspoon of bicarbonate soda to a glass of water. Think about your most-loved food for a few minutes until your saliva kicks in. Swig the bicarbonate soda and water back and if you're not belching like a drunk in 20 minutes you may need an acid recharge.

Your intestinal interstate

Once food has made it through passport control, and hopefully been sterilized, it enters the small intestine, where more digestive enzymes and juices break it down. If your belly balloons a couple of hours after eating then the enzymes in your small intestine may need a refill. The small intestine also sucks up all those lovely nutrients vital for health. Next it's on to the large intestine (colon). After absorption all that remains is the unprocessed food particles, fiber, digestive juices, dead bacteria, and water. The large intestine's job is to reabsorb the leftover water and make the rest into excrement.

Your intestinal interstate spans around 26ft (8m) or, to put this into perspective, if you rolled it out it would be as long as a tennis court. So you can see how, when compacted into your body, it's like a small twisty road, with tight corners and lots of places for food to get stuck. Processed and undigested foods in particular create traffic hold-ups. Living on junk may mean there is waste going back years in your system, making your intestinal pipes into a hazardous sewer. However, the great news is that by changing your plate you can rewrite your fate.

- -

☀ *Hot, Healthy, Happy: Spring-clean your colon*

The HHH 21-day diet is packed with fiber-, nutrient-, and water-rich foods that will polish your colon pristine and give you an inner glow. In a few days, I've seen clients turn their systems from crazy to calm.

- -

A-lister hotspot or Z-lister dump?

Ever waited in line for a trendy nightclub praying the doormen will let you in? The intestines operate a similar system. When you're hot and healthy your body's a top VIP hotspot. The nutrients are the glammed-up celebs with their stilettos and short skirts. Straight in, no questions asked. They make the place sexier, after all. Toxins, pathogens, and large food molecules are told to take a hike and keep walking.

Beneficial bacteria are your beefy doormen – they protect the body from invasion and keep everyone under control.[7,8] They produce antibiotic substances that restrain the baddies[9,10] – they even produce their own sexy nutrients. I want to give a big holler out to the top health-promoting guys, lactobacillus and bifidobacterium.[11, 12] We need these in the right numbers (about 85 percent of our overall bacteria) to stay exclusive. High-sugar diets, allergenic foods, the contraceptive pill, trauma, parasites, anti-inflammatory drugs, processed food, low stomach acid, constipation, stress, and even treated tap water can wipe out these guys in their millions.

If the beneficial bacteria end up down the toilet the pathogenic bacteria, yeasts, candida, and parasites start running the show. Unlike good bacteria they're sugar junkies and hooked on processed food, refined carbohydrates, and animal fats. Needless to say, things get scary fast. Before you know it, the nutrients are heading on out and pathogens, toxins, and large food molecules are littering up your pristine hotspot. If you've not been keeping yourself in tip-top shape then your body could be attracting the Z-list.

- -

☀ Hot, Healthy, Happy: Stop guessing and start changing

Consider a 'comprehensive digestive stool analysis with parasitology,' because this will give you an insight into your current levels of good and bad bacteria, yeasts, and parasites, plus a full breakdown of how well your gut is functioning. This test will arm you with knowledge, and knowledge is power. Make the right changes and take the guesswork out of it. Visit www.thefoodpsychologist.com to find out more.

- -

Is your health leaking away?

When the intestinal entry system is compromised it's a toxic implosion. Prescription drugs, junk foods, alcohol, sugar, artificial sweeteners, pathogenic bacteria, yeasts, parasites, and nutrient deficiencies all fire up inflammation in the gorgeous gut. The nightclub doorways get bashed in, creating large gaping holes in the intestine wall. A 'leaky gut' means undigested food pieces, waste particles, toxins, and pathogens start streaming into the body. Your beautiful body gets invaded, it's surveillance system (aka your immune system) screams panic, and immune complexes are formed. These travel to the liver, whose job it is to clean up the whole mess. As you can imagine, the detox capacity of the liver gets extremely freaked out and substances end up not being processed properly.

Soon there's a backlog of waste accumulating in the liver and fatty tissues. The toxins are stored as fat. Hosting a dumping ground, your susceptibility to infection, food allergies, Crohn's disease, celiac disease, skin problems, colitis, autoimmune diseases, and other 'allergic' disorders soar. Leaky gut has also been linked to inflammatory and infectious bowel diseases,[13–18] acne, psoriasis,[19] chronic liver disease,[20] and pancreatic disease,[21] as well as numerous conditions triggered by food allergies including eczema, hives, and irritable bowel syndrome (IBS).[22–26] Whoa, what a journey. You can see now why this incredible system is so vital to being hot, healthy, happy. If you want to look and feel fabulous then you need to create inner harmony in your gut. It's time to reveal the four-R formula for divine digestion. *Drumroll please.*

⚙ Hot, Healthy, Happy digestion in four simple steps

Following the HHH 21-day diet in Part IV in combination with this process will give you a gorgeous gut in no time.

Step 1: REMOVE the irritants

The HHH 21-day diet is perfect for combating nasty bacteria. This, in combination with natural anti-fungals (caprylic acid, berberine, garlic, plant tannins, or oregano, etc.), will eliminate pathogenic bacteria and yeasts. The anti-fungals you should take depends on the pathogens you want to kill. A 'comprehensive digestive stool test with parasitology' (CDSA+P) diagnoses the levels of both good and bad bacteria in the gut. If yeasts or pathogenic bacteria are found it will test different anti-fungals against them so you'll know which one to take to kill that strain. If the test finds a candida colony has taken up residence, check www.thefoodpsychologist.com for more information on combating the problem.

Now change your diet. The HHH 21-day diet is extremely gut friendly – it removes many of the common foods people are sensitive to (e.g. dairy, corn, wheat, soya/soy, shellfish, and red meat) and uses others in moderation. Still having a reaction? Then try removing eggs, citrus foods, nuts, and tomatoes. To be even more specific you could ask your medical practitioner to organize a blood-prick test for food intolerances. We also offer food intolerance tests at www.thefoodpsychologist.com that you can do at home.

Step 2: REPLACE enzymes and hydrochloric acid

Now it's time to kick start your food quarantine system. Digestive enzymes and stomach acid are your wellness *juju*, crucial for health. If you suspect you are low in these, take a good quality digestive enzyme, betaine, and pepsin supplement with your meals (not suitable for those with ulcers or gastritis), which will ensure the breakdown of proteins, increase assimilation of nutrients, kill toxins

continued on p.60

continued from p.59

and pathogens on your food, and reduce the risk of inflammation in the gut. Sipping diluted apple cider vinegar with meals, or using it in salad dressings, is also excellent for helping to break foods down.

Step 3: REINOCULATE with probiotics

With your system cleaned of pathogenic bacteria you'll want to bring some protection into your gut to keep everything in check. To do this, introduce a good quality probiotic supplement. Look for a supplement that boasts at least a billion live cultures.

Now you've rehired your doormen you need to remember to feed them to keep them strong and healthy, and their preferred food is prebiotics found in the following raw foods: chicory, Jerusalem artichoke, garlic, onions, leeks, asparagus, jicama, yacon, and bananas.[27]

Being low in prebiotics puts you at risk of the villains taking over.[28] Supplementing with FOS (fructooligosaccharides) is a delicious way to add prebiotics to your diet; it tastes like powdered candy floss. *Yummy!*

Step 4: REGENERATE the gut lining

Usually by this step the digestive system is operating smoothly and it is simply about healing the damage. Inflammation is a natural bodily process – it's designed to help the body heal. Supplementing with glutamine is an effective way of repairing the gut lining[29] and this, in combination with the good bacteria, helps keep your natural defenses strong. Those glammed-up nutrients will be heading on in any time now.

CAUTION: Always check with your medical practitioner before introducing supplements.

Hot, Healthy, Happy action plan

- ♥ If you suspect you may have pathogens and other villains running wild in your digestive tract then consider testing to find out what you're up against. Based on the results you could introduce a course of natural anti-fungals (e.g. caprylic acid, berberine, oregano, plant tannins, garlic, etc.)

- ♥ Follow the HHH 21-day diet, which removes many of the potentially challenging foods for the digestive system. In particular, get friendly with fermented foods (e.g. apple cider vinegar and cultured vegetables).

- ♥ Consider introducing a digestive enzyme supplement alongside your meals, and if you suspect low stomach acid then choose one with hydrochloric acid and pepsin.

- ♥ Rehire your nightclub doormen by introducing a good quality probiotic supplement and some prebiotics such as FOS.

- ♥ Finally, heal and repair your gut with gorgeous glutamine.

- ♥ Using the four R-formula (see pages 59–60) will give you a gorgeous gut in no time. Many imbalances – skin, hormones, or mood – stem from problems in the stomach and bowel so start by supercharging and healing your gut.

Chapter 4

Hormonal Havoc: Managing Your Monthly Madness

Mother Nature handcrafted our monthly rhythm to ebb and flow. She gave us food, an environment, and a lifestyle created beautifully to fit our natural design. It sounded good, but we got bored and busy. *Hello convenience, entertainment at a click, neon lights and rave dancing, microwave meals, drive-thrus, and 24/7 entertainment.* Modern life has given us a whole lot, but at what cost? The price tag may not say it but in exchange for modern-life products we've been handed hormonal mayhem. Before I give you the lowdown on the potential dangers of some of these chemicals, let's get hormone savvy.

The dating game

When we hit puberty our sex hormones estrogen and progesterone are ignited. If you want a life free of hormonal havoc, you need to be clued up on how these two play. Let me introduce your hormone controller, the hypothalamus. His job is to fire up your pituitary gland, to release two super hormones into your blood:

follicle stimulating hormone (FSH) and luteinizing hormone (LH), which create and release eggs from your ovaries each month.

The whole cycle is there to fix up your egg on a hot date with a strong swimmer. Let's assume you aren't going to be welcoming a bundle of joy in nine months. The egg gets stood up, no loving this month. The hypothalamus senses the egg's singledom and releases the first master hormone, causing the pituitary gland to release FSH. This hollers out to the ovary to churn out estrogen, the womb's interior decorator. She sets the scene, in case the next egg has better luck in the sperm department and gets some fertilization action. She spends around ten days plumping up the womb lining and breast tissue in preparation. Follicles are ripened and prepared in both ovaries. By day 12 the place is a love nest and estrogen is at the top of her game. At this point LH is released. On day 14 this surge of LH leads to ovulation and a mature egg is sent out from one of the ovaries ready for her big date. The egg then joyrides it down the fallopian tube, wafted along by hair-like tissues, cruising for some hot sperm.

The space left behind, once the egg is released, fills with blood and specialized cells. This is the corpus luteum, the factory site for estrogen and progesterone. If the egg doesn't get lucky then the corpus luteum breaks down and the blood vessels in the womb lining go into spasm. The lining sheds and here comes your menstrual flow. Estrogen and progesterone levels drop, signaling the hypothalamus to release the master hormone and the whole dating game starts all over again. Once estrogen and progesterone have worked their magic they head to the liver and then off to the gorgeous gut for elimination.

The case of the killer interior decorator

Now don't get me wrong, estrogen's a sweetheart. She gets your love nest ready for baby making, you can thank her for your breasts, curvy female figure, and vaginal secretions for comfortable sex. Your beautiful body needs her, but in all her natural glory. Nowadays we live in a sea of unnatural estrogens. Estrogen-like compounds called xenoestrogens ('outsider' estrogens) are in food, air, water, exhaust fumes, and plastics.[1] We eat, drink, breathe, and medicate with them. The body stores them as fat. Many toxins, such as dioxins, are lipophilic, which means they pollute the lipids and fats in the body, making us sick.

The trouble is, they're endocrine disruptors.[2] They all worship estrogen. Ever had someone hanging on your coat tails, trying to be just like you? That's exactly what estrogen is facing, a whole bunch of copycats. They trick the body and start mimicking her, stimulating the growth of the hormone-sensitive tissue. Talk about a case of mistaken identity. The poor body doesn't know what's hit it when it faces a combination of rogue fraudsters, natural estrogen, synthetic estrogen, and supercharged estrogens from food. It's a mixed CD of madness. The body spirals into estrogen overdrive, aka 'estrogen dominance,'[3] and estrogen is outcast as if she were a toxin.[4] Since even a little extra estrogen can spell disaster[5], it's hardly surprising that estrogen dominance has been linked to breast, uterine, and ovarian cancer,[6, 7] endometriosis, fibroids, premenstrual syndrome, obesity, migraines, and infertility.[8-10] The key to balancing your hormones is to know what you're up against. Let's give you a crash course on how to avoid these fraudsters.

The fraudsters

There are more than 100,000 synthetic chemicals on the market.[11] Some are in our food while others sneak in with pesticide residues or build up from non-biodegradable industrial contaminants. Once inside the body, these chemicals can scramble our hormones. We're genetically designed to adapt and go with the flow but these chemicals dupe our genes and can disrupt our endocrine and immune system. In combination with a lack of vitamins, minerals, essential fats, and phytonutrients (the hormone balancers), we're heading toward potential hormonal havoc.

💡 Beware: Worst offenders list[12]

★ **Phthalates:** Used in plasticizers (e.g. PVC, cosmetics, toiletries, etc.).

★ **Organochlorines:** Used in pesticides, especially DDT and Lindane (also used in insect repellents and pharmaceutical treatments for scabies and head lice).

★ **PAH (polycyclic aromatic hydrocarbons):** Product of burned or charred foodstuff; these are carcinogenic, so avoid barbecued meats, over-browned foods, etc.

★ **PCBs (polychlorinated biphenyls):** Primarily used as cooling and insulating fluids.

★ **Dioxins:** A by-product of many industrial processes involving chlorine (e.g. waste incineration).

★ **Toxic metals:** Mercury, cadmium, arsenic, lead found in deep-sea fish (e.g. tuna) and used in pesticides.

So how are these fraudsters doing it? Hormones are messengers. Your chemical FedEx girls, scooting round the body delivering info. They work hand in hand with our genes to make us healthy, vital, glowing, and fabulous. When they reach the cell they park up in the receptor site and deliver the message. For these girls to do their job they need a healthy little site to dock onto, which is why we need lots of lovely good fats (e.g. seeds, nuts, avocados, and cold-pressed oils) to create healthy membranes. A smooth flow of communication, from hormone to hormone receptor, to gene expression, to biochemical response.[11] This is how they groove, or should do, if these fraudsters weren't messing things up. Once in your body these chemicals mess with you in three ways.

1. They park up, blocking your hormone receptors so the FedEx girls can't get in.

2. They play dress up and pretend they're hormones.

3. They intersect messages, scrambling them.

In other words, they mess with our genes' ability to express themselves to our cells. The body is in new territory and just doesn't know how to deal with them. It's flummoxed.

A master fraudster: the contraceptive pill

Nowadays synthetic hormones are as much a part of being a female as a love of shoes: from menstrual pains to infertility and menopause, they're dished out as if they're wonder drugs and the answer to our prayers. *I say, label it what it is: the greatest human experiment.* Hormone birth control (whether it's the pill, patch, vaginal ring, or implant) is a master fraudster. It relies on the same synthetic hormones as HRT (hormone replacement therapy), which has well-documented problems including an increased risk of blood clots, stroke, heart attack, and breast cancer. Hormones in these pharmaceutical preparations are supercharged compared to our normal levels. Just like a fake designer handbag, they may look similar but they can't rival the real deal. A key that doesn't quite fit the lock. Jingle jangle, our biochemistry is being shaken. They block the receptor sites so the natural hormones can't work their magic. The fake stuff is also harder for the body to dump. It sticks around in our system, scrambling messages and wreaking havoc. Hardly surprisingly it has a spectacular list of side effects: irregular bleeding, high blood pressure, headaches, low libido, weight gain, sore breasts, vomiting, depression, nausea.[13] Long-term use has also been linked to an increased risk of cancer,[14-16] and thinning bones.[17]

As if that wasn't enough, did you know that odor preference affects who we're attracted to? Research has found women prefer men with a dissimilar chemical make-up (probably to avoid inbreeding). When you're taking the contraceptive pill your preferences shift: your body mimics pregnancy, making you prefer men with a similar chemical make-up to you. When you come off the pill you may not find that boyfriend is so hot after all![18] *Oh dear.*

So if they're not good for our health, why are we given them? Well call me cynical but pharmaceutical companies prefer synthetic hormones. After all natural bio-identical hormones can't be patented.[19] *Boom, boom.*

- -

☀ *Hot, Healthy, Happy: Make up your own mind.*

Your body is your queendom. You decide what to put into her. Contraceptive methods are a personal choice. Safe sex is crucial, but the contraceptive pill is not the only option, and it is perhaps worth considering other methods. I think if we really understood the implications for our health, fertility, and long-term survival then synthetic hormones would be ditched on the wayside. However, it is a personal choice and if you can't part with your method of birth control then you might find this easy two-step plan helpful in micro-managing the damage:

♥ **Hormone** contraceptives drain nutrients, so stock up on a multivitamin/mineral supplement high in magnesium.

♥ **Your** digestion can also be affected, so to keep that hotspot pristine, take a probiotic.

- -

Dirty dairy

Although the practice is outlawed in the UK and Europe, some US dairy farmers are reputed to pump up their dairy herds on recombinant bovine growth hormone (rBGH), which keeps the cows constantly on stork watch and producing milk. This artificial cocktail leads to another hormone, IGF-1. Some researchers suggest this is linked to the big C.[20, 21], although the jury is still out. IGF-1 is actually a normal part of all milk. It helps babies grow. In fact cow's milk is designed to grow a 40kg (90lb) calf into a 907kg (2,000lb) cow over two years.[22] Perhaps not the ideal chow if you want to rock those skinny jeans.

However, wherever we live, the simple fact is when we eat animals we eat their hormones. In fact around 60–80 percent of our estrogen intake is from dairy. But guess what? These are 100,000 times more potent than the environmental fraudsters. The truth is cow's milk isn't made for adult humans, it's made for babies, and in particular baby cows. We know this is true because between the ages of 18 months and four years we lose 90–95 percent of the enzyme lactase, which helps us digest lactose (the sugar in dairy). *Bloated tummies ahoy.* Undigested lactose is acidic, which spurs baddies to grow in our guts.[23] Finally, milk contains casein, which is nice and sticky (it's used as a commercial wood glue) and is a histamine releaser,[24] which is why dairy products can have us spluttering and sneezing. To protect itself the body produces mucus.[22, 25] Along with what Daisy is injected with to protect her from diseases, she also faces non-degradable PCBs, DDTs, toxins, and pesticides[23] that have built up through the food chain. In fact, even radioactive particles are found in milk.[26] *Bet that milk moustache isn't looking so sexy now!*

☀ *Hot, Healthy, Happy: Go dairy free*

The thought of life (or even 21 days) without dairy may feel a little overwhelming but don't despair, there are plenty of fantastic nondairy milks to discover. Try almond, hemp, quinoa, coconut, rice, or oat milk, which all have a delicious nutty flavor and taste great over some gluten-free granola. You could also trade dairy spreads for nut butters and coconut oil, although a little organic dairy butter on a baked potato won't hurt, as it's very low in casein.

Hot soya potato

The plant kingdom isn't immune to estrogen either. They have phytoestrogens. You'll find these in citrus foods, wheat, licorice, alfalfa, celery, and fennel. However, the big one is soya, and its hormonal effects are a hot potato in the health world. Studies suggest Asian communities have benefited from small portions of fermented soya foods. But like Chinese whispers, this has been translated by the Western world into the theory that we should be guzzling soya by the truckload for healthy hormones. Yes it's high in protein and cheaper than meat, but most of the soya is now processed, genetically modified, and heavily sprayed and supersized. It also contains phytic acid, which blocks the absorption of minerals such as calcium, magnesium, zinc, and iron.

So why is soya thought to be good for our hormones? Phytoestrogens lock into our little receptor sites. This blocks more toxic fraudsters from the environment getting in. It's been found to reduce the risk of developing cancer and reducing its reoccurrence. However, other studies suggest it promotes cancer growth[27] and suppresses the thyroid.[28] Confused? Well the jury is still out, but the bigger problem is that we are so overexposed to cheap, processed soya. It is cheap to produce and manufacturers fill out many foods with it. It is the same story for dairy. Our foods are packed with milk derivatives. We over-consume these products without even realizing it, because they are in everything from chocolate and oven meals to breads and ice cream. Finally, many people are unaware that they have a sensitivity to dairy or soya and suffer niggling health and digestive issues as a result. The HHH 21-day diet is the perfect antidote. It introduces a world of foods without all the extra junk.

- -

☼ Hot, Healthy, Happy: Be soya savvy

Stick with soya in its more natural form (e.g. edamame and soybeans). You can also enjoy fermented forms of soya (e.g. tamari, miso, tempeh, and natto). The fermentation process neutralizes the high levels of phytic acid and also has a probiotic effect which your digestive system will adore. Limit your tofu intake and combine it with mineral-rich seaweeds – tofu has been linked to brain aging.[26] Don't fall into the junk food soya trap and dump all the other substitute meat products, too, while you're at it; they're heavily processed, often contain dairy products, and can exacerbate digestive issues.

- -

Eliminating estrogen

Reducing your exposure to the fraudsters is vital but you also want to ship out that excess estrogen. In the next chapter you'll get a guided tour of your rehab center (aka your liver), where harmful villain-like toxins are packaged for elimination. Here excess estrogen is handcuffed to a conjugate called glucuronic acid, which escorts it out of your body safely, via bile and the gut to the toilet. Unless, of course, they're hijacked! Sneaky pathogens make the journey dicey. They produce a ruthless little enzyme called beta-glucuronidase who rips the glucuronide conjugate away from estrogen, setting her free to charge back into the body. After all the trouble of processing and packaging her up she's freed at the last minute! Screwy hormones and disastrous digestion are a sign this enzyme could be causing mayhem. The solution? Kill the villains, beef up your defenses, and supplement with the super nutrient calcium-d-glucarate. This will keep beta-glucuronidase in check and speed detoxification of estrogen and other environmental carcinogens. *Yippee!*

💡 Test your hormone levels

So how do you know whether your hormones are well balanced? Without measuring hormones, the treatment plan for recovery would be an educated guess at best, since levels can vary as much as 200–1,500 percent from person to person. For optimal balance it may be that only one needs adjusting, or several. Imagine trying to balance your bank account without your statement. Your body is no different. Hormone testing not only provides a basis for treatment but also indicates the precise imbalance. One of the best ways to assess hormone balance is by using a saliva hormone test called 'Rhythm Plus,' which measures estrogen and progesterone levels over a month, together with DHEA and testosterone levels. This can also include a measure of cortisol levels to test adrenal function. Visit www.thefoodpsychologist.com to find out more.

- -

☀ *Hot, Healthy, Happy: Eat up your greens!*

A high intake of cruciferous vegetables such as cabbage, cauliflower, broccoli, kale, and Brussels sprouts has been found to reduce cancer risk.[29] All these foods contain glucosinolates, which help prevent normal cells from being transformed into cancerous cells.[30]

- -

Adrenals: the CEO of stress management

So far we've met estrogen, progesterone, glucagon, and insulin. They're a few of our hormone posse. There's also thyroxin, which controls metabolic rate, cortisol, and adrenalin, which helps us respond to stress, and a whole bunch of hormones from the pituitary gland.

However, the adrenal glands are the CEO of our stress management. In the days when all men were hot Tarzan-like cavemen *(a girl can dream)*, our adrenals ensured our survival. Faced with the saber-toothed tiger they rushed our body's resources into 'fight or flight' mode. Run for the hills, or fight for our lives. Blood pressure rises, heart pounds, digestion slows, immune system kicks into action, adrenalin and cortisol flow. We're ready to whoop ass. Nowadays threats are rarely life threatening, but the adrenals are still drama queens. We tell them it's a disaster and they get into a fluster. Running late in stilettos, stuck in traffic, dropping your phone in the bath, angry bosses/teachers/parents, rumors on the Twittersphere, redline debt. The mind screams danger, and the adrenals panic. They also get whizzed-up on stimulants like coffee, sugar, and nicotine. If you soar from drama to drama, your adrenals will be in a tizzy. Over time they get overwhelmed, overworked, and exhausted.

☼ *Hot, Healthy, Happy: Go low GL*

Ever felt stressed off your head before your period? The reason is that progesterone, estrogen, testosterone, and adrenal-stress hormones are all steroid hormones made from cholesterol. So at your time of the month there's a greater demand for raw materials. You can feel all screwy and stressed out because your posse are competing with each other.[5] It's handbags at dawn. The HHH 21-day diet will help turn you from stress head to chilled chick. The magic remedy is low-GL foods and a stimulant shakedown. Pack out your diet HHH style with low-GL foods and you'll feel calmer and won't pack on the pounds each month.

Progesterone kidnapper

Now here's where this gets really interesting. Overworked adrenals can go hand in hand with progesterone deficiency.[3] If you're stressed then the adrenals churn out cortisol. To make this, they need pregnenolone and progesterone. When we're living from one catastrophe to another our adrenals struggle to make cortisol. Desperate times call for desperate measures. They take radical action and actually kidnap progesterone! Progesterone levels drop, knocking the estrogen to progesterone balance again. Pregnenolone levels also sink. This is bad news because we need her to make our anti-aging hormone DHEA, along with testosterone and estrogen. So you can see why keeping your adrenals happy is key to having hot, healthy, happy hormone balance.

☼ Signs of adrenal fatigue[31]

All of the following are signs that you may be suffering from adrenal fatigue:

★ Difficulty getting up in the morning

★ Poor memory

★ Fatigue after a good night's sleep

★ Craving for salt

★ Decreased sex drive

★ Decreased ability to handle stress

★ Increased time recovering from illness

★ Lightheadedness when standing

★ Mild depression

★ Less happiness with life

★ Decreased productivity

★ Increased PMS (premenstrual syndrome)

★ Decreased tolerance

★ Feeling better after evening meal

★ Mid-afternoon energy slump

★ Don't wake up until 10 a.m.

What imbalances the adrenals?

First, divine digestion and healthy adrenals go hand in hand. Bloating, indigestion, heartburn, and reflux all stress them out. An inflamed and irritated intestinal interstate forces the adrenals to churn out cortisol and perform damage control to reduce the inflammation. This is another reason to temper the road rage in your magical root system. Poor digestion = overworked adrenals = hormonal havoc.

Elevated cortisol actually destroys the intestinal lining.[31] Remember those nightclub doors? Well, too much cortisol bashes them in, which in turn causes more inflammation leading to more cortisol. This is a vicious circle. This is also true if you're living on a blood sugar rollercoaster; riding this also freaks out your adrenals. When blood sugar levels plummet the adrenals throw out cortisol and adrenalin to balance them. When they're overworked they can't produce enough cortisol or adrenalin so blood sugar continues to drop! Cue cravings, hypoglycemia, PMS, brain fog, poor sex drive, and excess weight.

In order to overcome adrenal fatigue, tempering the road rage on your intestinal interstate and jumping off the blood sugar rollercoaster are essential, as discussed earlier. Reduce your sources of physical stress (more on that in Part III), ensure you get seven to eight hours beauty sleep at night, and avoid over-exercising. Joint and back pain, and carrying excess pounds, all tax your adrenals, but following the HHH 21-day diet will soon have you jumping for joy at being able to get into those skinny jeans.

:ॐ: Do you have hamster syndrome?

Many people catch hamster syndrome in an attempt to shift the excess weight. They become hooked on pounding the treadmill. Like a hamster on a wheel they run, run, run, getting nowhere fast. This overworks the already stressed-out adrenals and keeps the body in breakdown mode. It's important to understand that our system is either rebuilding (anabolic) or tearing down (catabolic). To be hot, healthy, happy you need more rebuilding than tearing down. Adrenal exhaustion, chronic fatigue, and other chronic health problems are often found in a catabolic state. Cortisol and adrenalin are catabolic hormones. DHEA, testosterone, insulin, and growth hormones are anabolic. If we're running on cortisol and adrenalin then we're tearing things down and our health suffers. Punishing ourselves in the gym, living on stimulants, and running from one drama to the next prevents us repairing and rebuilding. We push and push, trying to drop the weight with sheer force; we ply ourselves with caffeine and other stimulants and forget the importance of nourishment. It's time to replenish and support your adrenal glands. They need love, too. The HHH 21-day diet will help you nourish your adrenals by reducing stress, balancing blood sugar, and supporting hormone and digestive function.

For some extra oomph you could consider some adaptogenic herbs (e.g. ashwagandha, Siberian ginseng, astragalus root, rhodiola rosea, and licorice root). Think your adrenals are flagging? Then take a saliva test called the 'Adrenal Stress Test' (visit www. thefoodpsychologist.com for more information).

Ignorance isn't bliss. Arm yourself with good knowledge and tip the odds in your favor. You have the power to protect, maintain, and improve your hormone health. The HHH 21-day diet is high raw, low GL, and plant based, making it perfect for balancing hormones. Your hormones and digestive system are interlinked, so it is vital to sort out your digestion, balance your blood sugar levels and manage stress. The sad truth is that it's impossible to eradicate hormone disruptors completely from our lives (after all, two million tons of phthalate is produced each year[32]), but we have the power to reduce our exposure. So take action now and start reducing the fraudsters in your life.

Hot, Healthy, Happy action plan

- ♥ Go organic and say goodbye to those nasty pesticides and herbicides in your home and garden.

- ♥ Up your plant-based foods and give Daisy a much-needed rest. The HHH 21-day diet is a plant-based, dairy-free diet so it should naturally reduce your exposure to estrogens in meat, soya products, and dairy.

- ♥ We now have a daily allowance for the plastic we eat. Crazy right? Impossible to avoid, but again reduce, reduce, reduce by avoiding processed meals and fatty foods packaged in plastic. Keep any edibles that are hot, liquid, or acidic away from plastic.

- ♥ Minimize liquid foods in plastic containers by choosing juice in glass bottles or unlined cans.

- ♥ Reduce your exposure to food in plastic. Use plastic food wrap sparingly. Opt for paper bags and remove food from plastic bags and wash immediately.

- ♥ Always remove foods from plastic for storage and never cook food in plastic; transfer foods into a ceramic container before heating.

- Don't eat burned and barbecued foods; scientific trials show that these are carcinogenic and should be avoided at all costs.

- Don't get caught up in the hype. Think carefully about the contraceptive pill and other birth control methods that secrete hormones. There are other choices.

- Use filtered tap water. Consider fitting a reverse osmosis filter made of stainless steel (not plastic or aluminum). If cost is an issue use a glass jug filter. Although this won't remove all the hormone disruptors, it may decrease your load. The best water is spring water bottled in glass.

- Use a chlorine ball in your bath. When you run a bath open the windows and let it run fully before going in. You can also get a filter head for your shower.

- Soak fruit and vegetables in water and vinegar, made by adding 1tbsp of vinegar to a basin of water. This will reduce some, but not all, of the pesticides.

- Opt for natural detergents wherever possible, use ecological detergents for washing dishes and clothes.

- Avoid bleached products. Wherever possible use unbleached versions, including teabags, toilet paper, and tampons.

- Switch to natural make-up, skin and hair products. There are now many wonderful online resources for natural beauty products – everything from lipstick and self-tan to shampoo and moisturizer. These are far superior in quality to those found on the high street.

Chapter 5
Beat Breakouts: The Formula for Supermodel Skin

For years I battled acne outbreaks. My face was a war zone of red lumps. I hid out in my house, cursing the mirror. Acne agoraphobic. My only survival tactic for braving public face time was trowelling on the war paint. The doctor armed me with lotions that could have stripped paint, and pills that had my body waving its white flag. Steroid creams, giant antibiotics, contraceptives. *Bang. Bang. Bang.* I also turned to the local beauty salon and traded my life savings for a room full of creams and face-burning facials. Hindsight's a b*tch.

Now I know better. Beautiful skin comes from the inside out. Contraceptive pills, antibiotics, steroids, toxic creams, did my body need more chemicals overworking it? I want to show you another way. Empower you with information that wasn't given to me. Help you make smarter decisions. Maybe it's not acne but occasional breakouts. Perhaps you're itching all over with eczema or psoriasis, or you just want to keep you skin firm and glowing. Whatever your skin scenario I know you want the formula for sexy skin.

Toxic rehab center

For clear and healthy skin you need to get toxin savvy and love your liver. All food and water, and the air we breathe, contain toxins. Inside you this very second, substances are being broken down, built up, and converted. Around 80 percent of this involves detoxifying dangerous substances, such as the fraudsters from the last chapter (see pages 65–69). Your liver is your body's rehabilitation center for nasty villains. The place where millions of dangerous chemicals are converted to harmless substances before being sent out into the world, shuttled through your elimination pathways. Toxic villains come in two forms:

1. **Exotoxins** are nasty rogues that enter your body in food, air, and water.

2. **Endotoxins** are made by the body with every breath, action, and thought.

The body's ability to rehabilitate these villains will determine how much damage they cause inside. If your body's rehab is overworked then your skin will become clogged and unhealthy!

As toxins move into the bloodstream, they're grabbed by antioxidants (your police officers on duty). They pick up the toxin, neutralize him, and escort him to your rehab center, the liver. Once the toxin is in custody in the liver, the antioxidant is released back into circulation, patrolling for more. However, if the liver is stressed out with too many toxic dropouts and not enough support, then the rehab center quickly becomes a halfway house. Skin problems, along with other debilitating symptoms (e.g. chronic fatigue, multiple allergies, frequent headaches, chemical sensitivity, hay fever, digestive problems, aches and pains), can all be a result of being overrun by toxins. Want to clear that acne, calm that eczema, or get a lovely glow? Then you need to understand how your rehab center works. Let me put on my tour guide hat.

- -

☼ Hot, Healthy, Happy: Up those antioxidants

Stuff yourself with antioxidant-rich foods such as cruciferous vegetables, citrus fruits, berries, and dark green leafy vegetables, seeds, nuts, and black beans. I love cherry juice: 30ml (1fl oz) of concentrate contains the same antioxidant level as 23 portions of fruit and vegetables! Oh, and it tastes delicious.

- -

Toxin rehab tour

Toxin rehab is a two-step process. Turning a toxic, drugged-up, nasty villain into a gentle and harmless substance occurs mostly in your liver by a rather complicated set of chemical pathways called biotransformation. This whole process happens via a series of enzymes reactions. Think of the enzymes as individual therapists and, in the rehab center, there are two therapy teams.

The first team of therapists, called P-450 enzymes, carries out phase one. Once they've worked with the toxin it's eliminated by one of three routes. Sometimes he is ready to leave the body straight away and is sent to the urine or sweat to be eliminated, or to the bile and leaves in your feces. However, some toxins need more work before they're harmless, and so are converted into intermediate compounds. But here's the thing, this actually makes them even more dangerous! The more villains that come into the center, the faster these therapists work to get them ready for elimination. But because the first therapy team sometimes works harder than the next, this can lead to a build up of even more nasties. Not great news for you.

The function of the P-450 enzymes depends on a long list of nutrients (e.g. vitamins B2, B3, B6, B12, folic acid, glutathione, branch chain amino acids, flavonoids and phospholipid, and antioxidant nutrients). So for this therapy team to work effectively they need a good supply of nutrients. But here's the thing: these enzymes will also use nasty substances to keep them going. A bunch of overworked therapists, they run on stimulants: caffeine, alcohol, cigarette smoke, exhaust fumes, high-protein diets, organophosphate fertilizers, paint fumes, saturated fat, steroid hormones, barbecued meats, and dioxins.

Phase two is more about building up than breaking down. This team takes the bad guys and sticks things to them to make them less harmful. A villain in a pink tutu? Okay not quite, but take over-the-counter painkillers, in phase two they have a substance called glutathione stuck to them, to make them less harmful.

So why does this matter? Because for clear healthy skin our rehab center needs to be in good working order. Our detox system is designed for a natural diet high in fresh, raw, and alkalizing plant foods. With a natural diet we have all the antioxidants we need to protect our body from oxidative damage caused by circulating toxins. We would also have all the nutrients our body needs to perform phases one and two of detoxification without overworking the therapists (enzymes).

The problem with modern-day living is that it exposes us to thousands of toxins, as discussed in the previous chapter. Instead of nutrients, food-like molecules trick the body into letting them enter. They wreak havoc, causing irritation and inflammation, and since toxins push their way through your skin, toxic overload spells beauty disaster.

Talk about toxin overload! The HHH 21-day diet will give your life and body a toxin overhaul. A spring clean if you will. Say goodbye and good riddance and give your rehab center a makeover.

☼ *Hot, Healthy, Happy: Support your liver*

If you want to love your liver, here are four steps to having a kickass rehab center:

Step 1: Dump trans-fats, HFCS, artificial sweeteners, and processed foods. They're packed with liver-damaging compounds. Instead stock up on organic fruits, vegetables, nuts, seeds, legumes, and spices.

Step 2: Supplement with choline, betaine, vitamin B6, methionine, folic acid, and vitamin B12, as these compounds are useful in promoting the flow of fats and bile to and from the liver. Eat foods rich in B-complex vitamins (e.g. oats, wild fish, leafy green vegetables, beans, and peas).

Step 3: This is optional, but you can also add milk thistle (available from health food stores), which protects the liver from a wide variety of toxins.

Step 4: Add turmeric to your food because it contains curcumin, which stimulates phase two.

Pesky breakouts

We all hate spots. So depressing. Everyone gets the odd one (always pre-date, right?), but acne is a whole other beast. Talk about a self-confidence killer. One in two people get acne, so if you're cursed with it then you're not alone. Acne affects the area of the skin with hair follicles: pores gets clogged with dead skin and fatty bits build up, creating a bacteria's dream home. Sebum is bacteria's food of choice: it moves in, pigs out on sebum and *voila*, acne!

So where does all the extra bacteria chow come from? You guessed it, our hormones! In fact, hormones called androgens ramp up oil production into hyperdrive[1], causing breakouts.[2] It may be that some women are more sensitive to androgens than others.[3] One androgen you'll have heard of is testosterone. If your diet is out of whack, testosterone converts to a more aggressive form, aggravating acne. Even if you're a woman, acne can still be caused by testosterone.[4] Excess testosterone can also cause mild depression, aggression, irritability, a deep or coarse voice, greasy hair, breast shrinking or male hair growth patterns. Well, the good news is that the HHH 21-day diet will address this problem. When your rehab center is supported and calm, androgens will be processed properly and not end up back in the blood where they move to the skin and start overproducing sebum.

However, for clear, glowing skin, progesterone and estrogen need to be in sync, too. As you know from the previous chapter, if these are out of balance you can get heavy, painful periods, sugar cravings, cramps, migraines, polycystic ovarian syndrome, and endometriosis. Growing up, I had all of these symptoms along with my acne, so I knew my hormones were off balance. The medical profession often prescribes the contraceptive pill or steroid creams for skin breakouts, but both remedies just add more toxins to the already-overworked liver; they may suppress some of symptoms temporarily, but they can manifest in the body in other ways. Obviously hormonal balance is strongly connected to liver function. The rehab center works tirelessly to process and package estrogen so it can be eliminated. For this we need lots of lovely nutrients and a strong, healthy digestive system. You can't have healthy skin without balanced hormones, a healthy liver, and a divine digestive system because they are all – say it with me – inter-freakin'-connected! *Cue Mexican wave.*

- -

☼ *Hot, Healthy, Happy: Limit animal and trans fats*

Limit your intake of animal fats and trans fats as these promote inflammation. Instead, enjoy raw plant fats from avocados, cold-pressed oils, seeds, and nuts. Essential fats are vital for healthy skin. You could also supplement with around 1000mg of EPA daily and some gamma linoleic acid. This will help to balance hormones and improve skin elasticity, and reduce inflammation in the skin.

CAUTION: *Always check with your medical practitioner before introducing supplements.*

- -

Divine digestion and hormonal harmony

Let's start with the link between acne and the gut.[5] How does the whole process go wrong? Well, as discussed in Chapter 3, if our food quarantine is on the blink, we can't break down protein (see pages 52–53). If our defenses are low (those trusty doormen) and the nightclub doors are bashed in, then there are a whole host of consequences for our health. Cue giant undigested protein molecules in the bloodstream, inflammation, leaky gut,[6] candida, low levels of good gut bacteria, and pathogenic bacteria. Old hormones and toxins will be reabsorbed and not processed properly and the whole thing just gets messy. Without soluble fiber (e.g. fructooligosaccharide/FOS), coupled with too much beta-glucuronidase running riot, estrogen is reactivated, messing with our hormone balance.

Greater bowel toxins and imbalanced hormones often result in acne. Other outcomes of inflammation can be eczema and psoriasis. Often skin problems are treated with antibiotics. Antibiotics don't just kill the bad bacteria they also wipe out our much-needed gut defenses. Since beneficial bacteria are vital for skin health,[7] killing them places us right back at the start again.

Certain conditions, such as leaky gut, mean that nutrients don't get absorbed and deficiencies of certain nutrients cause skin problems. In particular, vitamin A deficiency is a strong instigator of acne.[8] Many prescription medications are based on derivatives of vitamin A, which have a spectrum of harmful side effects from blistering to bowel damage (e.g. the contraceptive pill can lead to excessive levels of vitamin A by mobilizing liver reserves). High levels of vitamin A may explain why it helps prevent breakouts.[9] Moral of the story: supplementing vitamin A is not advised if you're on the pill but may be beneficial when coming off it.

CAUTION: *Vitamin A supplementation is not advised if you are pregnant or planning a pregnancy. Always check with your medical practitioner before introducing supplements.*

- -

☼ *Hot, Healthy, Happy: Make beta-carotene your BFF*

Increasing your intake of beta-carotene is a gentle way to improve collagen and elastin production, making the skin plump and supple. Top beta-carotene foods include carrots, spinach, sweet potato, kale, squash, apricots, broccoli, peach, and red pepper.[10]

- -

Along with vitamin A, it's thought that zinc could also be effective in treating acne[11] and eczema. During our teens we use up zinc during growth spurts. In addition, B complex (especially vitamin B6), vitamin B12, and selenium have all been found to be vital for skin. Want those lovely nutrients? Then make sure you eat them, or supplement them, and that your digestive system is strong and healthy so you can actually absorb them. Glammed-up, sexy nutrients only love pristine hotspots, remember.

You can also help your digestive system remove toxins by sweating. Your skin is your largest elimination organ, so when the body is overrun, it will try to remove toxins via the skin. Sweating heats up your circulation and helps secrete impurities, dirt, and toxins through your open pores.

- -

☼ Hot, Healthy, Happy: Love your skin

Take a good quality multivitamin with vitamin A (not advised if you are pregnant or planning a pregnancy), zinc, selenium, and vitamin E. An additional B-complex supplement may also be beneficial.

For clear skin start shaking that booty and getting on a sweat, or sweat it out in an infrared sauna. Kit yourself out with a one-person infrared sauna and you have an instant way of getting rid of those nasty toxins lodged in your body. Only about 1 percent of toxins come out in your sweat with a normal sauna but with infrared it's closer to 20 percent. *Whoa that's hot.* In fact infrared saunas are unsurpassed at shifting environmental junk out of your body.[12] Check out www.thefoodpsychologist.com for more information.

- -

The ugly side of the beauty industry

Who doesn't love delicious makeup, getting dressed up to the nines and looking at the top of their game? Like many women I grew up spending my money on every high-end cream and beauty product I could get my manicured hands on. Organic foods were one thing, but surely I didn't have to give up my favorite lipstick? After all, weren't natural beauty products for the hippy, tie-die fashionistas? Did my shampoo really matter that much? So I did some snooping and it turns out that most beauty products aren't so pretty after all.

The problem is that every day most of us are smearing our faces, washing our hair, and lathering our bodies with industrial chemicals: carcinogens, pesticides, reproductive toxins, and hormone disruptors. Most of us are not in the habit of sipping engine oil, yet here we are putting it on our lips, our eyes, or in the bath. And if you think about it, most of us use around 12 personal care products a day[13] so that's a lot of toxins for our systems to deal with.

💡 Chaos makers: What to watch for...

Parabens: Used by manufacturers to increase the shelf life of products, parabens inhibit enzyme activity, making them hormone disruptors. If you're buying beauty products, avoid those containing ingredients beginning with butyl, ethyl, methyl, or propyl.

Mineral oil and other petroleum-derived ingredients: These form an oily film over the skin to 'lock in moisture', and initially leave your skin feeling silky soft. However, locking in moisture also means trapping toxins and hindering normal respiration by keeping oxygen out.

Compounds (e.g. propylene glycol, alcohol, phthalates): These have been linked to decreased fertility in females and faulty reproductive development in male fetuses.[14] Commonly used in lipsticks, they also make nail varnish 'chip resistant' and allow hairspray to 'add flexibility'. But you won't find these listed on the label, they'll be elegantly disguised as 'parfum.'

Sodium lauryl sulphate (SLS): This detergent is found in approximately 90 percent of commercial shampoo, toothpaste, bubble bath, and shower gel; it's what makes things bubble and foam. Research has shown links to skin and eye irritation, organ toxicity, reproductive toxicity, neurotoxicity, endocrine disruption, ecotoxicology, and biochemical or cellular changes, possible mutations and cancer.

Remember the golden rule: If the label reads like a chemistry experiment, gingerly put it back on the shelf and run like a banshee.

Apart from the obvious gross factor in using chemicals on your skin, they could all be exacerbating skin conditions such as acne, psoriasis, and eczema. You also know from the previous chapter, that these chemicals wreak havoc on your hormones. Since the majority of breakouts are the result of an imbalance in your sex hormones, creating further problems by using creams and potions makes no sense. Masking the problem on a superficial level is in fact making the problem worse. Do things differently. Be a natural beauty not a toxic one.

☀ *Hot, Healthy, Happy: Be a natural beauty*

Go for natural skincare products that are free from parabens, SLS, and other nasties. Your skin and body will love you for it.

Hot, Healthy, Happy action plan

♥ Follow the four R plan in Chapter 3 (see pages 59–60) to ensure a hot, healthy, happy digestive system. Kill the bad guys running around your gut, replenish your beneficial bacteria, heal leaky gut, power up your food quarantine (replace digestive enzymes and HCL), and turn that body of yours into a pristine hotspot.

♥ With your digestive system in good working order you will be able to reduce the pressure on your lovely liver. You could also support your liver further by following my four-step plan to a healthy rehab center (see page 83).

♥ Drink plenty of water, and eat vegetables, fruits, seeds, and other gentle sources of fiber to keep your intestinal interstate free of road rage and topped up with sufficient skin and hormone healing nutrients. Dump the refined sugars and trans fats, and limit animals fats and dairy, which can be bad news for your skin.

♥ Eat foods rich in antioxidants that will help clean up your blood and transport more toxins out of your bloodstream for rehabilitation.

♥ Balance your blood sugar levels by dumping the refined carbohydrates and switching to low-GL foods. This, along with digesting your protein adequately, can help keep your cortisol levels down, which will have a beneficial effect on your hormones.

♥ Detox your life as much as possible by avoiding synthetic junk and toxins (parabens, etc.). What better excuse do you need to treat yourself to some fabulous new make-up and skin care products?

♥ If you suspect your skin issues are caused by hormone imbalances then follow my suggestions for boosting your happy hormones in Chapter 2 (see pages 37–50).

♥ Finally, consider taking a good quality multivitamin and mineral supplement that is rich in skin nutrients (e.g. zinc and vitamin A).

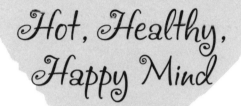

Part III
Hot, Healthy, Happy Mind

Chapter 1

Think Yourself Hot, Healthy, Happy

Have I convinced you that science makes you sexy? Boosting your biochemistry makes you red-hot: gorgeous skin and hair, a trim waistline, and skinny thighs. What you eat and drink makes you glow and shine, and gives you angel wings, but feeding your body beautiful isn't all green juices and superfoods. You only eat a few times a day, but you churn out a staggering 12,000 to 60,000 thoughts every day. You can dump the junk food, but if you're talking down to yourself, you're still feeding yourself rubbish. What you eat and drink is only half the story because being hot, healthy, happy is also about what's going on in your headspace.

Excess weight and niggling symptoms are everything to do with who we are, how we feel, and what's going on in our lives. Thoughts are unstoppable forces to be reckoned with, and they're the final spicy ingredients we're tossing into the hot, healthy, happy recipe.

Your mind is a sculptor. Every minute you shape your life by how you think. Want to supercharge your diet? Have healthy hormones? Clear your skin? Rev up your energy? Then pull on those cowgirl boots and lasso the power of your untamed mind. *PS: I'm going to show you how!*

☼ *Hot, Healthy, Happy: Let go of toxic beliefs*

Let go of your toxic beliefs about food and your body. Write down any negative beliefs you are holding on to and give yourself permission to let them go. Now that you appreciate the impact they're having on you, recognize how they're holding you back. Be kind to yourself. Give yourself time to grow, change, and adjust. The more you believe in your body's capabilities to look and feel how you want, the more chance you have of achieving it. I believe in you. Now it's your turn.

Declare your superpowers

Your mind and body are two peas in a pod. Stitched together with universal ribbon. Your body is hardwired to feel every Earth-shattering emotion. Over the moon or down in the dumps, your body can respond by bursting into tears. That rush of excitement when he texts you back. *Oh my!* The butterflies when you feel nervous at the prospect of facing a crowd or the red beamer when you mince your words. Thoughts and feelings create physical changes. You know how it works. But blushing, tingling, and running to the bathroom are just the tip of the iceberg. Your thoughts can impact your body in mind-blowing ways. Every little thought, feeling, and intention flows like an electric bolt through your body – changing it. Each one is so powerful that even your genes stand to attention.

What you think about your day-to-day life can actually switch certain genes on or off. *Wow, your mind is hot.* What an incredible ability, to be able to create your health and protect yourself from disease. If your beliefs can affect your biology then it's time to get your mind on your side, because it can dance and prance every single action in your body. Emotional hurdles manifest physical symptoms while positive thinking triggers healing. I'll let you in on a secret: your miracle mind has been curing aches, pains, and illnesses throughout your life without telling anyone. I think it's time you declared your superpowers.

Your cells have ears (well, sort of!)

Once upon a time biologists thought that our destiny was imprinted on our genes. Now that would suck because it would mean we don't have any control over our lives. Green juice, positive thinking, and fresh air would lose their sparkle, because our DNA would decide if we were hot, healthy, happy, or not. Thankfully, this theory had a hitch. Humans only have slightly more genes than a chimpanzee and a few more than a miniscule marine worm. We obviously bear no resemblance to either of these in the mirror – *it would take longer than a 21-day diet if we did*. So genes aren't the whole story. Scientists needed to peek beyond our DNA to understand how fascinating we are. Enter... *round of applause...* the hot science called epigenetics, which tells us that our genes are not our fate.

To understand the mechanics of this, we need to peer deep into our cells. What we see is that, instead of the nucleus (which holds the DNA), it is the cell membrane (the part surrounding the cell) that is the star player. Destroy the nucleus, the cell survives; destroy the cell membrane and it's cell Armageddon. The DNA is just a blueprint but the cell membrane is the manager. He holds the instructions. If the cell membrane is the middle guy, you may be wondering who is the boss? You guessed it... it's you!

What you eat, think, and drink whispers to your cell membranes, telling them what to do. Each one contains ravishing little receptors: tasty tuning forks that light up as 'signals' in the environment. These signals provide the instructions for effector proteins. What you eat and drink can make changes but the receptors also love energy fields. You may not know this but your thoughts create waves of energy and they also create energy fields. Therefore these telepathic tuning forks can read your mind. They then trigger proteins lighting up your DNA: thoughts transforming DNA, thoughts overriding biochemistry, thoughts changing your fate. Wow! That's awesome. You're in the driving seat, hot stuff. Your DNA is only a passenger. What you eat, drink, and think can flick those genes switches. Fall in love and genes turn on or off. Get a crazy idea, genes on or off. It seems you're not just along for the ride after all; you have a whole lot of power. You create you.

☼ Hot, Healthy, Happy: Polish up your inner chat

Notice what thoughts you are feeding yourself on a daily basis. Begin to tune in to your inner chat and polish it up a little. Are you nourishing your soul, or battering your system with junk?

Miracle pills

The white-hot truth: what you think about your body counts. Not convinced? Welcome... *drumroll*... to the placebo effect. Imagine you went a bit OTT on the cocktail therapy and woke with a pounder of a headache. You throw back some 'Extra Super Advance Cure-in-an-instant Painkillers' convinced they'll have you back in your hot pants in a flash. Chances are the pain will lift. You assume it's the magical chemical formula but in reality you could get the same relief from a jellybean. You just need to believe it will work. I'm not messing with you. Research has demonstrated this time and time again. You tell your body this pill will heal you and it takes you at your word. This is the phenomenal placebo effect.

A placebo is the fake designer bag of the drug world: a dummy medicine with no fancy pants chemical healing powers. Medical trials use them to prove whether drugs work or not because placebos are not supposed to heal. To fool the mind, a placebo has to be identical to the real thing. If the drug being tested is a yellow pill with a red circle, then the placebo must be dressed up the same. That pretend drug is a miracle healer though. Even without the fancy chemicals it zaps its healing *juju* and cures anywhere from 10 to 100 percent of people.[1] The unsuspecting patient believes they are taking medicine; they believe they will heal, and *voila* what do you know... they do! Mmm, now I wonder how many people taking the real deal would actually be cured by the placebo effect? Ever wondered why a treatment works for one person but not another? *Belief baby, belief!*

Now back to your hangover. Someone beat you to the last expensive painkiller and you're left with the cheap own-brand ones. Not convinced? Then they probably won't work. Even doctors are clued up on the power of what we think. Drugs are usually dished out when they're the 'in thing.' Once a new shiny drug appears then the earlier one loses its sparkle. The formula is the same but the belief has left town. This isn't to say that drugs don't create physical changes or heal ailments; they do, but so does your mind. What you think matters.

Molecules to emotion

So how does all this mind–body stuff work? Let me introduce you to your neuropeptides. Brain whiz Professor Candace Pert nicknamed these 'our molecules to emotion.[2] To get your head around this, picture a child's shape-sorter toy. Correct shape... you get a direct hit and it flashes, and this is how chemicals get groovy with the brain. They all have their own racy receptors. They slot in and ding-dong, the body switches a function on. Your thoughts light up different areas of the body. That 'gut feeling' telling you something's not right is due to experiencing real chemical changes in your gut. Specific neuropeptides light up the gut receptors, giving you that sixth sense. You get asked out, hear exciting news, get a brilliant idea, and you can literally feel your body tingling. This is your neuropeptides fitting into those parts of the body – your mind creates physical feelings. Think back to those painkillers, which work by locking into your pain receptors. If you were convinced that the jellybean was the undiscovered healer then your body would believe you and produce its own natural neuropeptides to fit into your pain receptors, just as if you had taken a pharmaceutical preparation. Either way, you would be fresh faced and feeling clearheaded in no time.

Healthy eating maniac

Foods and drinks are not immune to the placebo effect either. Eat for your body type, blood group, raw, vegan, vegetarian, paleo, high protein, low protein, etc. I thought my head would explode with the myriad of 'right' ways to eat. The truth is that food obsessions are bad news. How often have you launched into a new orbit of healthy eating, navigating your journey using a 'this food bad, that food good' mantra, only to end up confused and freaked out?

At the start you feel on top of the world but by dessert you're overwhelmed with advice. You become a healthy-eating bookworm, devouring diet plan after diet plan. Now you're cringing in horror at how you once rolled. In your clueless days food hadn't done much harm, but now you know about all the additives, preservatives, flavorings, fat, calories, and sugar there are more foods to slip up on than actually eat! Something 'forbidden' sneaks in and your brain hits the mental torture button. **Your body hears every single thought.** It takes a mental beat and your cells are flooded with unhealthy signals.

So, having stuffed this book with healthy eating information I want to reassure you that food obsessions are not part of the HHH 21-day diet. Forget overwhelm and perfection. Snap off that angel halo, it's weighing you down. Focus on eating highly nutritious food but don't beat yourself up for flirting with forbidden foods when the mood takes you. Your body will survive. It can cope. Stay out of the stress response. Heads-up: don't give yourself a double whammy of a chocolate cake and junk food thoughts.

- -

☀ *Hot, Healthy, Happy: Killer donuts*

Write yourself a permission slip to let go of toxic nutritional beliefs. *If you don't, I will!* Just stop thinking: 'Food is the enemy,' 'Fat makes me fat,' 'My appetite is out of control,' 'Once I lose 14lbs (6kg), I'll be happy,' and so on. This thinking is unhelpful and links food, something that should be good for you and pleasurable, with suffering. *News flash: You are not being attacked by donuts; chocolate cookies won't assassinate you while you sleep.* Food is not the enemy. Post-It Note this to the fridge: 'Food makes me fabulous.'

- -

What about emotional eating? Does it scare you? Been there. You're an emotional being: a juicy, deliciously complex, unpredictable, wild creature. You laugh, cry, cheer, break down, and fall head over heels in love. Emotional eating is inevitable. Get over it. We love food. It feels amazing. Your emotions are going to pull up a chair at the table so make space for them. Striving to assassinate emotional eating is just a way of avoiding uncomfortable feelings. It's camouflaging deeper stuff. It's your body nudging you and saying: 'Hey you, something's going a little nuts in here, check this out.'

While we're here let's clear something else up. You don't have a willpower problem: 'If only I had more willpower, I could stop camping out in front of the refrigerator.' Forget this nonsense. We usually overeat when we're stressed out, distracted, overwhelmed, and in dire need of something to soothe us. We don't stay present, think about the food, the tastes, enjoy each mouthful, and allow it to nourish us. We wolf it down so fast our brain is left in a daze: *Whoa. Hold up. Wait. What just happened? Did I eat something?* Slow down. Increase your awareness. Expand. Savor every mouthful and you'll say goodbye to overeating.

☼ *Hot, Healthy, Happy: Be a conscious muncher*

Before you eat something ask yourself: 'What will this do for my body, mind, and immune system?' Make eating a conscious, mindful choice, not a mindless activity.

You're a natural superstar

Getting fresh with natural whole foods is a show of self-love. Love you and you make loving choices; it's not a challenge, restriction, or chore. A healthy body slurps up healthy food. The stress response is deactivated and you radiate at a higher vibrational level. When you're zoned out, calm, and chillaxed then whole foods and healthy habits become your idols. They make you a rock star. Things just fall into place, so don't stress out. No one (not even me) goes from chocolate sandwiches to green juices overnight. Far from it, your body and mind will adjust and change gradually. Lean into it. Dip your toe in. Your body will adapt.

Convincing yourself to be healthy, and strictly avoiding certain foods, is short-changing your body's incredible ability to be naturally healthy. Chastising yourself about eating chocolate, while scoffing your preferred bar of confectionary, just creates stress. Food obsessions support the idea that your body is vulnerable. You're incredibly strong. You're designed to be hot, healthy, happy. When you live with ongoing symptoms, excess weight, and the blues this can slip your mind. Think about the last time you caught a head cold. It passed, right? No big deal. You had a headache. It just lifted. Maybe you broke a leg robot dancing in your Jimmy Choos. Once it was set it would have healed all by itself. You're naturally programmed to heal and reach your superstar potential.

- -

☀ *Hot, Healthy, Happy: Relax into it*

You're custom made to be unique and vibrant. Unhealthy foods and toxins pose far more of a risk if you ignore emotional signposts, or when you're lost and bewildered in the stress response. Your thoughts are powerful. What you think about food and your body matters. It's about what you eat, drink, *and* think. So chill out, relax, and focus on being happy.

Cruise in the hot, healthy, happy zone. Don't make rules, instead bend and flex like a Zen master yogi. Eat, drink, and think for energy, clear skin, healthy hormones, and a confident mindset. If you're emotionally and physically powered down, you'll be more vulnerable to making bad food choices and nasty toxins.

- -

When I was sick I kept my diet squeaky clean, but nowadays I take a more chilled approach. Hot, healthy, happy isn't a dogmatic way of being. It's a VIP invite to conscious choices. Listen to your body. You're the creator of your life. Experiment and find your own groove. We're all different. Trust your instincts. You're in charge so own your choices. If you're going to pig out on chocolate cake then sit back, put your feet up, own your power, and enjoy every single delicious bite. Then get right back to taking care of your body and giving it the right fuel to shine.

Hot, Healthy, Happy action plan

♥ Let go of any toxic beliefs you may have about foods; forget trying to eliminate emotional eating and give up worrying about lacking willpower. Instead, focus on staying present and eating consciously and mindfully.

♥ Declare your superpowers. Your mind affects your body. If you want to be hot, healthy, happy then dump the junk talk and polish up your inner chitchat.

♥ What you think about what you eat counts. Forget perfection and instead focus on stocking up on goodness. If you find yourself winking at naughty delights then forgive yourself and move on.

♥ Surf in the hot, healthy, happy zone. Don't create rules around food that you know you're going to break. Instead, listen to your body and focus on giving it what it needs. You create you, so own your choices.

Chapter 2
Go With the Flow: How to Float Through Life With Ease

Relax, chill, let go, live in the now. Sounds great in theory, but for a stress junkie this might sound like mission impossible. I've been there, too. Juicing, okay. Salads, easy. Give up stress. *You're kidding, right?* I was running on that stuff. How could I possibly have time to juice, prepare foods, take supplements, and do all this cleansing without going at 100mph? Meditation. Isn't that for monks? *Stop thinking for 15 minutes, err... my brain won't go for that.* Being a perfectionist, and overly competitive, didn't exactly go with laidback. I remember the fateful day I saw my adrenal stress test results. The look of disbelief on my practitioner's face was a picture: stage four adrenal fatigue, or put another way, completely exhausted adrenals by 20 years old. *What could I say? I'd been busy.*

Stress: HHH saboteur

Stress is addictive. Overwhelm is our second nature, and we seem to take comfort in chaos. Our poor adrenals suffer as a result and have us heading for disaster. Research has linked stress with almost every major illness. It eats us alive. If we want to shake off the excess weight, skin breakouts, digestive problems, or hormonal havoc, we need to break up with stress. I promise you the world won't crumble into a zillion pieces if you learn to chill out a little. It isn't mascara; you can definitely live without it. So release and let go, because stress is the ultimate hot, healthy, happy saboteur. What you eat and drink play a role, but what goes on in your lovely brain is vital. Your thoughts are like a Thigh Master shaping your body every single day. Running late? Missed deadline? Lost car keys? How you react is the definer. Stinking thinking is junk food to the mind. Stress makes us sick. Disease is actually dis-*ease*: negative thoughts and stress. If you want to look and feel fabulous then grab your passport, because I want to smuggle you out of the stress zone.

Stressed out, the clock tortures us. We feel lonely and overwhelmed. Our awareness shrinks and we can't see past our problems, barriers, and struggles. Fear is designed to keep us alert and alive. We separate ourselves so we can karate chop danger. If we live constantly in stress mode then we see ourselves as separate from the world. Disconnected from others and the awesome universal energy within and around us.

Fight or flight: this is our survival response for life-or-death situations. Nowadays it is less saber-toothed tiger and more annoying ex; less starving to death and more overeaten on Ben & Jerry's; less lost in the wilderness and more lost on Facebook. Other than the odd spot of nasty turbulence, we're rarely terrified for our lives. Even when life or death moments crop up, our body recovers *tout suite*. We go from 'OMG, even the flight attendant looks freaked out!' to 'Wow, it's hot. Beach time!' That's how we rock. Fight or flight panic then... *I wonder if that comes in pink?*

Stress doesn't live in the beautiful present

If we were stressed only when it really *was* life or death, life would be sweet but who are we kidding, most of us spend our days driving ourselves nuts. Stress sucks, but it rarely lives in the here and now. We're tormented by 'should haves' or 'what ifs.' We get worked up over things that happened years ago, things that haven't happened yet, and events that may never happen! Nowadays stress lives mostly in our heads. We're terrified of criticism, losing control, wasting time. We bulldoze through daily exercise, work round the clock, shop till our feet ache, and write 'to do' lists longer than the phone book: multitasking, worrying, anxiety, panic... *argh*. Living in the stress zone has us swimming in a sea of stress chemicals and teetering around in our stilettos in exhaustion! Why are we so stressed out?

- -

☼ *Hot, Healthy, Happy: Breathe baby*

Breathe into your belly. We spend so much time sucking in our tummies. When you're alone loosen that top button, breathe deep into your belly, focus on your breath and nothing else, and give your internal muscles a little well-earned massage. This is being mindful; this is living in the moment.

- -

Crazy consciousness

There are around seven billion people on the planet, yet we still feel lonely! Huh? How often have you hit a party feeling like a loner, yet rocking it on your lonesome, feeling happy and at ease? It isn't really about other people, is it? Wellbeing comes from feeling that crazy connection to the blue sky, Earth, and stars. Feeling at home sweet home in the world. Our brains are incredible, but they mess with our happiness. Wired to interpret everything around us as separate, we feel alone, fearful, and dare I say, stressed out. This is just surface reality. Just how we see it. Everything looks fixed, solid, and material, but that's not how it really is and I can prove it, so listen up.

If you have a bookshelf like mine then you'll have read the word 'consciousness' a gazillion times. If not, don't fret because we'll soon get you up to speed. Consciousness is having awareness of your thoughts, emotions, memories, sensations, and environment. It's always moving and grooving. In fact, let's face it, most of the time we have brain diarrhea: non-stop streaming and shifting thoughts, feelings, and sensations moving at breakneck speed. Right now, for example, I am typing this thinking about the words to write: *Wow this chair is hard and man I'm thirsty I need a Coke (got ya!)*. Consciousness creates your world; it shapes your physical reality and body. *Wild, I know.* Your magical mind creates physical changes, even affecting what happens in the world. Sounds crazy but to really get to grips with this, let's dive into the sexy world of quantum physics.

Quantum physics rocks

Super-smart physicists tell us everything is energy; our material world is simply an illusion, created by our phenomenal brains. If this is a little too Keanu Reeves of *The Matrix* fame, bear with me. Your iPad, this book, the sofa are all just energy. Your body? That's just energy, too. Thoughts and emotions? You guessed it superstar – energy. There are visible forms of energy you can touch, hold, and throw around and invisible ones such as your Wi-Fi connection, radio waves, microwaves, and electromagnetic fields.

I wake up, turn on my radio and Lady Gaga is singing in my kitchen. In the past (before you read this book obviously!) you popped dinner in the microwave and 'ping' it would get all warm and toasty without your eyes seeing anything happen. Power up your laptop and you can Google 'The Food Psychologist' and tune in to my rocking videos. *Thank you, Mr. Invisible Energy.* And we accept all these invisible forms of energy as being perfectly normal. Most of us don't understand how these work; in fact scientists still don't fully understand how and why electricity works, but we rely on this energy to make life sassier.

Invisible forms of energy are everywhere, and we know this is true because most of us get irate when they go haywire: for example, when our phone can't get a signal. Pink, black, or diamante, it doesn't matter, your phone is a structured and visible energy system interacting with electromagnetic waves. Your body is similar. It's a structured and visible energy system interacting with thoughts, emotions, and a universal energy field. In other words, your thoughts and emotions are simply forms of energy. Just like the box nuking your food, the electromagnetic waves are letting you Google. You're holding this book or eReader, and you can taste that cold glass of green juice *(cue lip-smacking sound)* because your brain is brilliant at interpreting complex vibrational frequencies. Don't be fooled, the world is not how it looks. Everything is energy, and energy is inseparable, including your thoughts, emotions, and consciousness. When you get your head around this whopper, the whole game changes.

There is no 'you' and 'not you' to your body and the universe. When you go deeper into quantum physics, you find only one whip-cracking energy field. Don't take my word for it. Trust those über-intelligent quantum physicists. In the 1920s they began to look at the teeny tiny parts creating our world, as if they were opening up a Russian doll. Peering closer and closer, they found that there is no solid stuff. They found absolutely nothing! Instead of smacking their heads for time wasting, they were awestruck and named nowhere land the 'quantum field.' What this tells us is that only waves of energy exist. Think about that. If there's no solid stuff, there's no real separation between anything. You and the chair, you and me, you and Robert Pattinson *(ooh tiger!)*: you and the universe are meshed together by an energy field flowing through everything. Everything around you is created from the wondrous quantum field. This means that at a basic level everything is consciousness. So if, for example, you have a diseased organ, at a deeper level of reality this isn't some inanimate organ, it's simply consciousness. This is why visualization can be used to heal disease and the body. This may also be why we can flick genes on and off with thoughts and emotions. Mind and matter; making love at a quantum level.

☼ Hot, Healthy, Happy: Tap into your natural power

You have the most incredible power at your fingertips. There's a whole lot of life force surging through everything you do, think, and feel. This energy field guides the growth of your body. Hot, healthy, happy, or sick and miserable? Your consciousness decides. You can choose to resonate with your world. You can even create your physical reality. Thoughts and emotions are part of your consciousness, and this determines what comes into existence. What appears as real and solid. We live in an amazing, conscious universe. You create your world and I create mine. We're not helpless victims, we're creators. This is an inevitable and incredible part of living in a conscious universe. We can use this to heal our bodies, find a hot date, and even make our dreams come true. It all starts with what you think. Everything in your life is created from the inside out. You're the commander in chief. You decide. Did you realize that kind of power was within you? So tell me, what do you fancy hustling up?

Tip of the iceberg

To feel connected to everything, we need to wave goodbye to stress. We can only do this by a shift in perception – by seeing everything, including ourselves, afresh. This is how you become a miracle maker. Imagine this incredible universal energy field as a huge ocean of calm and free-flowing waves. With our headspace in stress land, we see ourselves as a tiny droplet of water – separate, solid, insignificant, and disconnected from everything around us: this is everyday thinking for most of us. We get tricked by our conscious mind and see ourselves only in our physical form. Of course, your conscious mind's a superstar. After all, you can thank her for all the moving, singing, dancing, and chatting you do, but this only makes up 3 percent of your mind. What on earth are you doing with the other 97 percent?

Let's give a round of applause, and if you're feeling like it, a standing ovation, for your subconscious mind, who outdoes herself. She's in charge of most of your bodily functions. It doesn't matter how awesome your memory is, if you actually had to remember to breathe, pump your heart, blink, etc., you would have lasted five minutes. Fortunately, she keeps you ticking, moving, and grooving without you ever giving it a second thought. Think of your mind as being like an iceberg floating in the icy, blue water. You only see the tip: your conscious mind. As a result, we assume how we think is just chemicals firing in the brain. Oh no, sexy lady, there is a whole lot more going on under the hood. You're a vital part of a much bigger universe; the trees, stars, mountains, and it's all connected to you.

- -

☼ Hot, Healthy, Happy: Listen to what you're feeding your mind

How much of your day is spent feeling stressed out? Listen to the thoughts you're feeding yourself. When you begin to feel stressed, take a moment to ground yourself: breathe deeply and focus on the present moment – what is happening right now. Notice how often you feel like a wave, and how often you feel like a droplet. Make a conscious choice to shift into wave mode as often as possible.

- -

Go with the flow

Most of us spend our lives feeling stressed, lonely, and insignificant. We feel scared, overwhelmed, and worried about our fate in this big, crazy world. We think the only way to stay safe is to be perfectionist control freaks. We criticize ourselves, blinkered to the good, and sometimes only see how we and everyone else is messing up. But in reality, you aren't separate. You're plugged into an incredibly powerful energy source. Life is free flowing, just like that beautiful ocean. Yeah, you may be a little droplet of water, with your beautiful self-identity, but you're also part of a far greater energy field. Shifting into wave-like consciousness can help you feel part of this amazing power. It moves you away from the stress response to a more chilled place where you go with the flow.

- -

☼ Hot, Healthy, Happy: Stay loose and flowing

Letting go can be tricky. But there's no need for black and white and plenty of room for shades of gray. You don't have to be either stressed or chilled, you can pull up a chair happily somewhere in the middle (say, 40 percent droplet and 60 percent wave). The more you stay loose and flowing, the more your body and mind will thank you.

- -

The more you're in the hip and happening space – the present – the more you're plugged in to your higher self: best buds with the universe. Not only are you more chillaxed, you also get a VIP pass to universal knowledge on demand. Ever heard of the collective conscious? It's like the internet for our minds. We all have our computers (our personal subconscious and conscious mind), but with the right equipment we can access other information.

When a new thought arises, or ideas are formed out there in the world, it's like a new blog post is being uploaded. Our subconscious doesn't change, but the intelligence of us all shifts ever so slightly. New information becomes available to access. This is why information travels at lightning speed. It often doesn't need to be read or heard – everyone just intuitively knows it. We connect with our ability to intuitively interact with other energy fields – physically, emotionally, mentally, and spiritually. Sure, we can read stuff in books and newspapers, but intuitively we already knew it. For example, history records show that new discoveries, inventions, or eras of creative renaissance often appear in one culture and then spring up elsewhere shortly afterward, without the two having any form of communication. How often have you been able to anticipate the words or actions of someone else; been able to tell what they are thinking or feeling, or seen things through their eyes? Or perhaps been thinking or speaking about someone and they call, or you then run into them? I can't count the number of times I've picked up the phone to call my mother, only to find her on the other end of the line, having rung me!

Guess what, when you're hooked up to your higher self, answers and opportunities appear as if from thin air. In this zone you feel safe and loved. The stress response is switched off, as is fear. In this space your body can heal, and intuitive messages fly around like hot cakes. So connect to the universal energy and become a force to be reckoned with. Gain access to information your rational mind can only dream of. Get hooked up with your intuition and obtain the power to shape your life any way you desire. Become limitless. Time, bountiful. Feel connected to everything around you. In this place you don't lose you, but become part of something bigger. Life becomes effortless. You feel joyful, creative, forget problems – become Miss Solution Finder. You feel whole. This is the hot, healthy, happy mindset.

☼ *Hot, Healthy, Happy: Stay grounded*

Next time you feel stressed, take a big, deep breath and remember that you are part of a far bigger universe. Give yourself a moment to feel that incredible power you have behind everything you do. Ground yourself. Take off your shoes and walk in the dirt. Feel the wind in your hair. Repeat to yourself: 'I am safe. I am loved.'

Self-love comes before skinny jeans

What you think about your body, your life, and your world matters. It shapes everything. Becoming hot, healthy, happy begins with the thoughts you feed yourself. This doesn't mean we can live on pizza and fries *(nice try though)*. You're still a physical being. You need nutrient-dense, whole foods, beauty sleep, and heart-pumping exercise, but you need to stop the talking down to yourself: cursing and chaos. Stress, junk food, and stimulants are a tightknit gang. Fast fixes and fast foods are quick, cheap, and easy. That constant stream of stressful thoughts like 'I never have enough time,' 'I'm not getting anywhere,' 'Life is so hard,' 'I never have any money' make junk foods and stimulants the perfect solution. When we are time poor, exhausted and overwhelmed they feel like the magic remedy. They drug us out of our body. Help us avoid issues. Silence the body's cries for help. We ignore what our body is saying and push through because we think there's no time to really look at what is going on for us.

☼ *Hot, Healthy, Happy: Stay present*

Focus on the 'now', because stress rarely lives in the present moment. Listen to what you are feeding yourself with your thoughts. Dump the junk. Think healthier, happier thoughts and a hot, healthy, happy life will follow. If you struggle to change your diet and lifestyle, it is likely that you are still hanging on to old thinking patterns and limiting beliefs. Help your body move out of the stress response by giving yourself a break. Take a moment. Breathe. Go with the flow.

Once you're able to step out of the stress response, the world opens up. You suddenly have time to prepare food, prioritize your health, look after yourself, and invest in your wellbeing. So you can see there is a formula for success. To fit into those skinny jeans you know you have to change your diet and way of living, but to do that, you must first make an emotional shift toward self-love. It's not the other way round: 'When I have more time...', 'When my skin clears...', 'When I have more energy...', 'When my backside is smaller...'. We place so many conditions on our happiness. Switch it up. Turn the tables. Do it the other way round. Change your thoughts first.

We think if we can get skinny then we'll love ourselves. Believe me, it doesn't work that way. You must first change how you think. You could be on the best weight-loss program in the world, but if you're in stress mode your body won't be in the right physiological state to lose weight. So be kind to yourself – patient and loving. Give yourself time to grow and progress. Your body is simply a mirror of your mind. Change your thoughts and you really can change your life.

Hot, Healthy, Happy action plan

- ♥ Ditch the ultimate hot, healthy, happy saboteur – stress. It is time to escape to a more chilled and relaxed way of being.

- ♥ Stress rarely lives in the here and now, so focus on staying present. Drop 'should haves' and 'what ifs' from your vocabulary.

♥ When you feel alone, disconnected, and fearful, remember that this is just surface reality. Don't let your conscious mind trick you. At a deeper level everything is connected by one big energy field, so focus on that feeling of connection by imagining yourself as a free-flowing wave, as opposed to a little droplet.

♥ You resonate with your world. Your life reflects your thoughts, so choose your thoughts wisely, starshine.

♥ Instead of beating yourself up for eating unhealthy foods or not exercising enough, begin by focusing on stepping out of the stress response. Once you feel more relaxed the world will open up, and you will have more time to prioritize your health and body. Remember, fast food is the perfect food for fast-paced, stressful living. Change your thoughts first. Repeat this mantra: 'I have plenty of time.'

Chapter 3

Growing Up Unprotected: How to Build Strong Boundaries

Let's talk boundaries. Are you suffering a boundary breakdown? Then don't be surprised when you look in the mirror and see the following plastered across your forehead: 'Here for your convenience. Your lifetime/ambitions/dreams/desires/whims [*delete as appropriate*] are far more important than mine.' It is said that when you don't show people how to treat you, you show people how to treat you. To be hot, healthy, happy you need strong boundaries. Healthy boundaries make us like Sleeping Beauty in her stone tower: chilled, snug, and secure. Without them we're driving around with our taxicab light on, just asking for people to take us for a ride.

Hold up! One minute you're saying we need to get connected with everything and now you're saying we need boundaries. What's the deal? It might seem like a paradox, but look closer. Boundaries separating parts of a whole are vital. That little droplet with its own sense of self can surf those calm, loving waves. Every part needs to work independently to keep the whole caboodle hot, healthy, happy. Everything needs clear boundaries and purpose in the circle of life. The healthier your boundaries, the more you live with sparkle and swagger. The more you shine.

Boundaries can also be tricky. They are invisible shape shifters that change with time but, like your fingerprints, are completely unique to you. Before you bail and page skip to visualizing your dream life, hold back, because mastering boundary building is the key to a hot, healthy, happy life. Boundaries define the communication, behaviors, and interactions we accept: fabulous, healthy relationships or toxic ones? Your boundaries decide. So grab your hardhat and start rebuilding.

Strong as Superwoman

Boundaries are the little black dress of the universe; everything in life needs them to survive. Cells need cell walls. Energy waves have vibratory differences. Boundaries protect our sense of individuality: they keep enemies at bay while letting our friends snuggle in close. Think about your beautiful body. If your blood gets contaminated, it can't keep you pristine and glowing. Toxins, stimulants, parasites, and yeasts will rampage those nightclub doors and your body chemistry will go nuts, sending your cravings into overdrive. Destroying the whole can easily be achieved by striking off the smaller parts first. It's a takedown, piece by piece.

Healthy boundaries make you as strong as Superwoman, because when you can say, 'No, thanks' to the things you don't want, it leaves space for 'Yes, give me' to the ones you do. Safe and secure, we're a force to be reckoned with. We believe in our superpowers. Forget bottling up frustrations and then exploding when we're shaken too hard. We own our power and inspire other everyday angels to grow their wings and fly. You're unique and radiant. You've a responsibility to care and protect yourself. Here's the struggle: see that priority list of yours? Your name goes first. 'Put me first? You must be crazy.' That's right. Always secure your own oxygen mask before helping others.

💡 Different types of boundaries

Both physical and emotional boundaries are important. No half measures; both are vital. Physical boundaries keep you safe. Someone stands too close – eek, you feel invaded. You step back, they move closer. 'Back off buddy, you're crowding me!' *Setting boundaries. Delicious.*

Physical Boundaries
Here are some examples of how these can be violated:

★ Getting uncomfortably close to you. Creep alert.

★ Touching you inappropriately when you don't want them to. Give them the smack down and shout it from the rooftops.

★ Reading your texts, e-mails, letters, diary, files, etc. Passwords, people, passwords.

★ Invading your space – you know, like barging into your room without knocking. If you can't padlock them out, make sure you let others know when you need some privacy.

Learning to stand up for yourself is one of the greatest, juiciest gifts we can give ourselves. So throw a bow on it and sign the card: 'To Wonderful Me, because I'm worth it!'

Emotional and intellectual boundaries
These keep your self-esteem strong and help you separate your feelings from the feelings of those around you. Without these, other people's tiffs and tantrums can throw you into a whirlwind. Here are some examples of unhealthy emotional boundaries:

★ You give up your plans, dreams, and goals to keep others smiling.

continued on p.118

---

continued from p.117

★ You find it difficult to separate where you end and others begin. You let their moods determine your happiness.

★ You play the blame game and pass your problems on to others.

★ You feel responsible for other people's feelings.

★ You often tell others how to think, feel, behave, etc.

Power up, princess

Hot, healthy, happy chicks need boundaries, self-respect, and integrity. Otherwise the door is ajar and unwelcome guests can walk in with their mucky shoes. Unhealthy boundaries make us vulnerable to emotional pain, codependency, depression, anxiety, and physical illness. We can't live life on other people's terms, or let others run our lives for us; and trying to run someone else's life isn't healthy either. Think about it, what did you want to be before the world told you who you were?

The problem is that we're sponges to others' beliefs. Sadly, most of us miss the lessons on the laws of nature, the power of attraction, positive thinking, listening to our body, and creating our lives from consciousness. Instead, we allow others who are lost and bewildered to lead us. We've followed their lead and become strangers to our higher selves. The path back may be overgrown, but it still exists. Hunt for the obstacles holding you back. You're here, aren't you? You showed up. That means you have spark. Acknowledge your strengths and champion your life. Cheer yourself on. Believe in your abilities. Stand up for your life. Boundaries equal self-respect.

- -

☀ *Hot, Healthy, Happy: Polish your inner and outer shine*

Think about it: how can you respect others when you don't respect your own shining light? Simplify your life: what others think about you is none of your business, because you can't control how they feel or how they see you. What others think is oh so complicated; it is based on their childhood, their demons, heartache, happiness, ego, and dirty laundry. You don't need to know that stuff. Trust me. You've got your own stuff going on, so leave them dancing their own tune. Instead, focus on polishing your own inner and outer shine. Glow with positivity, joy, contentment, and kindness; it'll dazzle them and draw them in. Be warned though, these qualities can't be faked. A pure, loving, and divine spirit only shines from a hot, healthy, happy place of self-respect. So just start and power up, princess.

- -

Are you rocking healthy boundaries?

Signs you have super-hot boundaries:

- ♥ You feel assertive and confident when giving your opinions, thoughts, feelings, and needs. 'Yes' and 'No' are both in your vocabulary, and 'Sorry, I'd rather not' is locked and loaded for the occasions when something isn't right for you.

- ♥ You don't freak out when others say 'No.'

- ♥ You keep your needs, thoughts, desires, and feelings separate from others around you.

- ♥ You love making healthy choices.

- ♥ You take responsibility for you.

- ♥ You have wickedly high levels of self-esteem and self-respect.

- You share personal information gradually when you're in a relationship.

- You feel confident about protecting your physical and emotional space.

- You know how to take care of your needs.

- You share responsibility and power with those around you.

Signs your boundaries are wearing thin:

- You're terrified of saying 'No' in case you're rejected or abandoned.

- You people-please and struggle to work out who you want to be.

- You feel you have zero power to make decisions in your life.

- You struggle to protect your physical and emotional space.

- You always feel responsible for other people's happiness.

- You often find yourself saying, 'Okay, that's fine,' when you really want to scream, 'No way!'

- You struggle to be assertive and to communicate how you feel.

- You say 'Yes' because you're afraid of conflict.

- You feel stressed and overwhelmed by life.

- You feel spiritually, emotionally, and physically sucked dry.

- You spend time running about after others and leave no energy for you.

💡 Do you need a boundary rebuild?

If you need a boundary rebuild, start by getting clued up on your values. Every action you take fulfills a value: either moving you toward a desirable feeling or away from one that is not so hot. Once you know your values you have a yardstick against which to assess your behaviors, habits, and communication. If they don't measure up to your values, then they need to change.

So how can you discover what you truly value? Start by writing two lists: one with the feelings you want to feel and the other with those you don't. Go for those you can create. Don't choose feelings you can only get by someone else acting in a certain way. For example, 'I value feeling secure' as opposed to 'I value being attractive to so and so.' Once you have listed all the things you do and don't value, prioritize the attributes on your values list.

Imagine you have a magic wand that could give you any of your values. Which would you choose? That becomes the number one value on your list. Now keep going until you reach six or seven values that reflect who you are. It might include attributes such as honesty, kindness, authenticity, punctuality, etc. Take a good look at each of them. Ask yourself:

★ How do my values make me feel?

★ Are any of them out of date?

★ Am I hanging on to someone else's values (e.g. a parent, teacher, partner, etc.)?

Scrub those values that no longer fit you, or are based on other people's priorities. Find out what is really important to you. Once you know your values, you'll immediately recognize when either you or someone else tries to undermine them, and this knowledge will help you to create stronger boundaries.

Staying positive

Beware, boundaries bring tricky choices. Beliefs, behaviors, events, and life plans will threaten them. How often have you declared, 'I am going on a diet' only to have someone offer you a tray of pastries? Or decided to give up alcohol just when you're invited on a big night out? Maybe you decide 'No more kissing bad boys' just as the one who broke your heart declares he has changed. *Of course he has!* Stay on track. Bring out the heavy armory. Sucker-punch. When you feel weak, don't invite them to pull up a chair. You're a smart cookie. You know what'll throw you off balance. What ignites your spark and what drains your life force? With practice, your judgment will become crystal clear.

Ready to stake those energy vampires? It's impossible to be hot, healthy, happy when your emotional and physical energy is being sucked from you. Open your eyes. Notice what's going on. Do you have one of those so-called friends whose life is always spiraling from one drama to the next? Someone who only calls you when they need something? Are you constantly running around after the people in your life and never getting anywhere in your own life? Truth-test it: why have you tolerated this for so long? Can you feel it? Start gluing the pieces of yourself back together. All those parts you've split up within yourself as you took on other people's ideas, beliefs, agendas, stories, and BS. Trust yourself as your consciousness grows. Expand. Reflect. Revamp. *Now you're getting close to self-love.*

A word of warning: as you become clear on who you are and what you want for your life, other people might have a hard time accepting this new fabulous you. Give them time to discover the more authentic you. As you shine out confidence and happiness, they'll start shining back. Your universe mirrors your internal world. If you're irritated and fed up, this is what you'll see in the world. Smile, radiate, and ooze joy, and the world will reflect this back. Like attracts like. So if those around you challenge the fact you have changed, stay strong, wellness warrior, keep your integrity and don't waver – if you fold now you will lose not only their respect, but your own. You'll crush your confidence in your abilities. That would be heartbreaking.

Ninja Barbie

Where do you need a boundary rebound? What about that crafty credit card? No more maxing it out when life feels a little dull. Do you want to stop arguing with your nearest and dearest? Perhaps you want to stop people-pleasing to avoid conflict. Get comfortable with creating waves. It makes life more interesting, you'll see. Start cutting the ropes, breaking free, and escaping whatever is strangling your life force. Don't destroy fixable relationships, but get honest about what's polluting your life.

Creating a body and life you love begins by first recognizing what to remove from it. This doesn't have to be a negative experience. Instead of thinking, 'Little Miss M. drives me crazy, I'm so sick of her moaning,' try instead: 'I just love being around Little Miss H., she is such a sparkling star. I want to make more time for her in my life.' Making space for the hot, healthy, happy people in your life leaves less room for toxic relationships. If the doomers and gloomers need to stay in your life, keep it short and sweet. Don't invest your precious life energy in them. Create some super-hot boundaries and let go of anyone who breaks them down.

If, no matter what, you're stuck with the negative people in your life, then get Ninja Barbie on them. Never lose sight of what their issues are. Don't let their issues dirty your crystal waters. Don't get sucked into the drama. Listen, but give up the need to control, because your advice isn't going to shift them. Let go and breathe. Acknowledge your limits. Stay strong and hold firm. Always keep in mind the people who really matter, the things that fill you with joy, light, glitter, and stardust. Danger stamp whatever takes that fairy dust from you.

☀ Hot, Healthy, Happy: Leave room for the things you really want

If you're struggling with the 'No' word, remind yourself that by saying 'No' to something you are saying 'Yes' to something better, something you actually want. Accept that you can't do it all and pick what works for you. In this way you build your self-confidence and esteem, and other people will respect your boundaries.

Bad food breakup

Breaking up with bad food habits is all about boundaries, too. How often have you tried to become healthier and happier by focusing on what you don't want? 'I'm not going to eat cake any more,' 'I'm going to stop drinking coffee.' Honestly, who are you kidding? Your subconscious mind doesn't understand negatives. What it hears is 'I am going to eat cake' and 'I am going to drink coffee.' So switch it round. Always focus on the positive. 'I'm going to have a green juice every morning.' *Ah, now we're talking.* 'I am going to eat more raw plant foods.' Sure, you'll probably have some coffee and even some cake later, but the truth is, the cleaner your system becomes the less these foods will make sense to you.

As you lean into the HHH 21-day diet you'll find that your taste buds and sensitivity shift, too, and suddenly that massive piece of chocolate cake and cappuccino doesn't seem so mouthwatering anymore. All you can think about is how you'll feel post splurge – jangly and bloated. Before you know it, you're craving a glass of green juice and a few slices of mango (*yes, really!*) This is what it feels like to eat intuitively, to trust your body to know what it wants.

In the same way, if a toxic relationship or bad habits just won't shift no matter what you try, then get honest with yourself. Ask: 'What am I holding on to? What is keeping me from putting my body's needs first?' Whether food or friends, we can hang on to things for longer than we need, but perhaps it's time to say, 'So long now!'

☀ *Hot, Healthy, Happy: Exorcize what is non-negotiable*

To build hot, healthy, happy boundaries start by exorcizing those things that are non-negotiable. Make a list of all the things that you just aren't going to waste your delicious life force on anymore: relationships, behaviors, habits, etc. Now get emotional. Feel each one. Work through the list and let that inner voice of yours bellow, 'FROM NOW ON I WANT TO _____!'

As you do this create a picture in your mind of that situation. See yourself having positive relationships, eating well, and being hot, healthy, happy in all areas of your life. Connect with how it makes you feel. Notice where it links to in your body. And when you're ready, manifest it in your life; write it down or declare it out loud: 'FROM THIS DAY ON, I WILL [*fill in the positive action*] TO CREATE THAT IN MY LIFE.'

Hot, Healthy, Happy action plan

- ♥ So you reckon you have this boundary business down? Keep asking yourself: 'When push comes to shove, can I put me first?' I hope so. Stand up for what you want, and be a creator not a follower.

- ♥ When you clear the junk from your body, mind, and environment you make space for the good stuff. You can finally go after what you want from your life.

- ♥ We all need hot, healthy, happy boundaries. They equal self-respect.

- ♥ Instead of focusing on the foods you don't want to eat anymore, the activities you don't want to be involved in, or the people you want to distance yourself from, think about what you want more of in your life.

- ♥ Discover what makes you sparkle and what drains your life force. Be honest about the relationships in your life, and begin to notice who simply takes, takes, takes. Maybe you need a relationship revamp.

- ♥ Get comfortable with creating waves. Remember, saying 'No' leaves space in your life for 'Oh, yes!'

Chapter 4
Your Inner Three-year-old: How to Heal the Child Inside

I am standing on the beach naked. *That's right, butt naked.* My hair is long, blonde, and wild. I have a crazy look in my eyes. My skin is slightly torched from the sun: a sticky mess of seawater, sand, and sun cream. I'm dancing, jumping, skipping, and running in and out of the water. Waves crash against me. I'm singing and laughing with utter joy. Here is the thing: I'm not alone; in fact, people surround me. The best part? I don't care. It doesn't enter my mind who is looking or what they think. Lost in a wave response, I feel connected with the powerful sea, sun, and sand. I've forgotten my past. The future isn't of interest. Present. Free. In the now... I am three years old.

Over time, things changed. She learned to quiet her voice and worry: people are staring; sit still; avoid hurt and pain by 'acting appropriately'; and shrink down to save others' egos. That appearance changed her opportunities. Criticism stung. Her heart could be broken (and it was, numerous times!). She bent and accommodated. The out-of-tune singing was saved for the shower, the dancing and skipping for gym time. She saw that her body wasn't perfect after all. There was a lot to think about. Control became a priority and strategizing the 'what ifs' an everyday pastime. She heard she should learn from her mistakes – there were stacks. It was hard work going through them all each day. Soon there wasn't time to be happy-go-lucky anymore. Eventually she just forgot who she was.

Are you all grown up?

Most of us start out carefree: completely in love with our sparkling, amazing selves. Connected to the universe, wave response on tap. As we grow, things shift. We shift. We shape ourselves to our environment and other people. Things go wrong. We blame ourselves. Parents get angry or upset. We wear responsibility. We discover 'if only.' If only we could do things right our parents would be happier/love us more/not punish us. If only we were thinner. If only we were smarter. It's difficult. We feel faulty. Not good enough – imperfect and guilty. We learn to pretend. Fake it till we make it. Look happy even when we feel crushed inside. We learn scripts to make sense of our world. Ways to cope with dysfunction. We create false beliefs about our lives, our selves, our bodies, and our world.

Over time we tame and control that wild, childish side. Creative and chaotic becomes structured and organized. Emotional and sensitive becomes controlled and detached. Happy and joyful becomes sophisticated and task-oriented. We tell our inner child to be responsible, serious, and grown up. It's too much pressure for her, so she crawls inside us and hides herself away.

She is still there, you know? Hiding out in your subconscious mind. Sometimes you let her come out. Perhaps when you're having so much fun you forget yourself? You laugh and roll around, enjoying frolicking, frivolous nonsense. What about crying at weepy movies? Riding rollercoasters? Sneaking on the trampoline when no one's watching? Skidding down the grocery store aisles on your knees? No? *Oh right, that's just me then.* Surfing, swimming, or throwing some serious shapes on the dance floor – there she is.

Your inner parent

It isn't just your inner child in there. She's not living alone, because our inner parent supervises her. Listen in. Is she being offered loving, supportive, kind, encouraging words? 'You are such an awesome girl,' 'I really love you,' 'You're so incredible and thoughtful,' 'You're good enough just as you are.' Or is it more like this: 'You're doing that wrong,' 'What will so and so say,' 'You are so useless, can't you get anything right,' 'Why are you always late? You're so disorganized!' 'You can't wear that. Look, you have back fat!' Yeah, thought that might be the case. Informing child protection about her evil ways right now, aren't you? Perhaps it's time to send your inner parent to parenting classes? Replace the nagging with encouragement. Criticism with kindness. Anger with love. Change the stories she tells and the words she uses.

Here are some inner parent loves:

- ♥ You have the freedom and power to make your own choices.

- ♥ Do what you want to do. You have my permission to be 'selfish.'

- ♥ Always make time for the things you want to do.

- ♥ Choose who is part of your life. Keep those who make you feel sparkly, and forget those who bring you down.

- ♥ Live and love harder.

- ♥ Give yourself time to enjoy your achievements.

- ♥ Remember, you have all the time you need.

♥ Laugh, sing, dance, play, and have fun every single day.

♥ Use seriousness and inflexibility as your cue to inject some nonsense.

♥ If you're sad, cry. If you're hurt, share it. Let it all out.

♥ Allow yourself to be vulnerable.

♥ You don't always have to do things for other people.

♥ Allow others to do things for you.

♥ Make your own rules.

♥ Make happiness, joy, and excitement the cornerstones of your life.

♥ Let yourself feel sad, anxious, upset, and worried – as long as you share it.

♥ Come up with solutions; it's okay if no one else agrees.

♥ Take risks and make mistakes.

♥ Let your imagination run wild.

♥ Be honest with yourself.

♥ When you're angry, be angry.

♥ Make your own decisions.

♥ Love and be loved by someone.

Unfinished business

We humans have ridiculously long childhoods *(and I'm not including the 30-year-olds who still take their laundry home!)*. But this makes us very dependent on our parents. Survival means tuning in to their emotions, thoughts, beliefs, and feelings. Hints of disapproval, criticism, rejection, and separation are bad, because they trigger our fight or flight response, while unhappy or disinterested parents equal a threat. Kids are easily traumatized. Sensing danger or helplessness means trauma. Being hit, criticized, scolded, screamed at, shouted at – 'You spoiled brat,' 'You stupid child,' 'You're such a pain,' 'Just behave,' 'Eat everything on your plate or you're not leaving the table,' 'Stop being a crybaby' – just creates fear, fear, fear. Self-esteem gets bashed, confidence dented, and unhealthy stress chemicals flood the body.

Our beliefs are often based on our parents' beliefs. So our consciousness can come from them. Beliefs shape our health and happiness. They can flick genes on and off. *Whoa! That really gives a whole new meaning to inherited conditions doesn't it?* We didn't learn from what our parents said, but by tuning in to their emotions and watching their reactions. If your childhood was filled with tension and stress, this is what you learned. Your body may now exist in constant stress mode. Any little thing and your system hits the panic button. Maybe you're living on hyper drive, surviving from achievement to achievement. Drama to drama. Frozen in the fear response. Running on autopilot. Sleepwalking through days.

Until we are seven years old, our conscious mind is under construction. Events we're unable to process properly are sent straight to the subconscious. Think of your subconscious as the ultimate hoarder. Throughout your life she shoves every little keepsake, lifetime experience, belief, event, and fear into her giant magic memory box. Everything is downloaded, counted, and filed away. With your conscious mind in development, any trauma you experienced was stored away without being worked through and resolved. Those beliefs became your truths and they tell you how to perceive future events. Perhaps your mother was always obsessing over her weight, so you concluded that having a perfect body was vital. Maybe your parents were always rude and disrespectful to each other. Perhaps you learned that it's normal for one parent to talk down to the other, and it should just be accepted. You then may repeat these patterns throughout your life.

- -

☼ *Hot, Healthy, Happy: Replace old beliefs with shiny new ones*

Work out who and what you want to be. Don't place limitations on yourself. Just dream. How would you like to feel? Now work out what you would need to believe about yourself for this to happen. Start replacing your old beliefs with these new shiny ones.

- -

We all love to be right. Our brains are actually programmed to help us. They work by using our perception to guide our choices, and everywhere we go we look for evidence to prove ourselves correct. So negative, faulty beliefs become self-fulfilling. Are you hanging on to negative childhood beliefs? Then it's likely you're walking, talking, living proof that those limiting beliefs are true. If we grow up holding on to these kinds of notions then our emotional maturity gets stunted. Change your beliefs and the evidence will change with them.

Bogus beliefs

You know it's time for an overhaul if any of the following beliefs ring true with you:

- ♥ Life is hard.
- ♥ I'm not good enough.
- ♥ To be loved, I need to be perfect.
- ♥ The world is a dangerous place.
- ♥ I can't trust anyone.
- ♥ I need to keep my feelings hidden.

- ♥ I need to stay in control to stay safe.
- ♥ I need to pretend to be happy, even if I'm not.
- ♥ Love hurts.
- ♥ I'm unlovable.
- ♥ I'm insignificant.
- ♥ I'm an idiot.
- ♥ I'm a failure.
- ♥ I'm useless.
- ♥ Everyone always leaves me.
- ♥ No one ever notices me.
- ♥ There is no point in trying.
- ♥ I can't change my life.
- ♥ I need to put other people before me.
- ♥ If I say 'No' I'll be rejected.
- ♥ Nobody understands me.

Your scared inner child

When we take dysfunctional beliefs from childhood into adulthood, our inner child is left with a bushel of unfinished business to deal with. Perhaps you grew up too fast? Were you a little 'mother', or did you take on responsibilities as a carer? Maybe, instead of 'overly responsible', you opted for the 'overachiever' label. You learned how to put on a happy face or repress your happiness, passion, or feelings. If you weren't given the chance to mature, your inner child could still be waiting to grow up. There could still be a scared little three-year-old inside you. You can still feel her fear though – her anxiety, worry, or panic over silly things. Maybe when these feelings come up you deny them. Perhaps you feel you need to hide them to live up to others' expectations.

Maybe you cover up the real you. You wear a mask, always trying to look good and be good but opening up to others is a terrifying concept. But here's the thing, the longer you keep your inner child hidden, the more problems you can face.

What happens when you ignore your inner child?

Below are some of the consequences of ignoring our inner child:

- ♥ Always feeling out of place.

- ♥ Being unable to have fun, plan, relax, and deal with stress.

- ♥ Working all the time (possibly even a workaholic) instead of appreciating life.

- ♥ Needing to achieve in order to feel worthy.

- ♥ Feeling guilty no matter what we do, because we just don't feel good enough.

- ♥ We take ourselves too seriously.

- ♥ We don't enjoy spending time with family.

- ♥ We can't understand people who live for enjoyment.

- ♥ We hide ourselves away in case people find out we are inadequate.

Healing past pain

We all have past pain, that's life. But to accept all of ourselves we need to heal by loving our inner child. Love is a phenomenal healer: it can flow down deep into our most heart-wrenching memories and illuminate the darkest, murkiest corners of our mind. Only you can change your thoughts. Only you have the power to make new choices. Only you can choose to think differently. Forgiving and loving your inner child opens doors. The universe is watching your back, so it's time to reconnect with your beautiful inner wild child. Show her how to grow up into a hot, healthy, happy girl. Love her. Appreciate her. Praise her. Give her lollipops and kisses. Skip with her. Do the hula-hoop. Sing out loud with her. Do handstands in the street. Every day, tell her she is perfect just as she is. She needs you to cheer her on. She deserves to hear that you love everything about her. Even the parts that did all the crazy, stupid things, the parts that were strange looking, the parts that were daft and foolish, and the parts that messed up. Every single part of ourselves. Just as we are.

☼ Reconnect with your inner child

Begin by getting into a relaxed state. Make yourself comfortable and focus on your breathing. Take nice big breaths into your belly. Breathe right into your stomach, giving your internal organs a little massage, pushing your belly out; then exhale, letting your belly relax. Breathe all the way in, then push the breath all the way out. Keep a gentle rhythm. Become aware of any tension in your body; relax your shoulders, shift if you need to, and release any tension. Breathe into any tight parts. Start with your feet and then move up to your thighs, stomach, chest, and shoulders and down your arms. Breathing into each area releases any stress and makes you aware of the energy in your system. Release, let go, and notice how calm you feel. Finally, spread this warm, relaxed feeling throughout your body until you feel peaceful.

See your inner child
Now picture yourself as a little girl, anywhere between the age of three and eight.

★ Watch how you interact with your family. Are you happy, joyful, carefree, energetic, excited, and loving life? Or are you serious, sad, unhappy, disappointed, scared? What was life like for you as a child?

continued on p.136

continued from p.135

★ Imagine yourself at school. How do you play with your school friends? How do you get along with them? Notice how much fun you had and what you enjoyed doing.

★ Watch yourself in the classroom. Notice how you are around your teacher and being in school.

★ Can you only see an unhappy little child? Then try to remember your last happy experience as a child. This is your inner child who has hidden herself inside.

Listen to her

Once you've identified your inner child, grab yourself a beautiful journal and start jotting down answers to the following:

★ How would you describe your inner child?

★ What age were you when your inner child went inside?

★ What made your inner child hide away?

★ What have been the negative consequences of ignoring your inner child?

★ How can you tell when your inner child comes out to play?

★ Looking back, what irrational beliefs did your inner child have about life?

Are you willing to deal with these, and replace them with the truth? If you want to feel free and happy you need to deal with these. Then your inner child will feel safe enough to come out and play. Ask your inner child:

★ What messages does your inner child still need to hear that were left unsaid?

★ Is your inner parent happy to give these messages to your inner child?

★ Are you ready to enjoy the little things in life?

★ Are you ready to make time for fun in your life?

Hot, Healthy, Happy action plan

- Your inner child loves nature, so take a walk in the woods, run on the beach, and soak in the sun, moon, stars, and sparkles. Breathe deeply. Slow down. Let go. Laugh. Eat tasty foods. Savor each moment. Dance. Chill. Be still.

- Start enjoying the small things in life. Have you forgotten how gorgeous the natural world is? Draw, paint, or photograph it. Get out of bed and catch a sunrise. Listen to the birds sing. Get down in the dirt and grow some delicious veggies. Take in the sights, sounds, smells. Touch and explore.

- Begin to notice how you feel. Journal your days and explore your inner world. Go on an expedition in your mind and seek out new feelings. Throw on *Legends of the Fall* or *The Notebook;* grab a box of tissues and have a sob.

- It's important to notice the good things that happen every day. What makes your heart sing? Daydream. Play more. Dump guilt. Make fun non-negotiable. Freewheel through playtime and forget the rules. Make wild and carefree your defining characteristics.

- Forget judging eyes: if they knew what was good for them they would be rolling around with you.

- Abandon artificial stimulants: you only need alcohol and drugs when your inner child's in hiding.

- Send your responsible self away somewhere for a while – a distant country, or the moon.

- Fall in love with your incredible imagination. Laugh, cheer, jump, bounce, cartwheel, roll around, hula-hoop, have a food fight, water fight, throw snowballs with your friends.

Invite your friends' inner children round and play pin the tail on the donkey, bobbing for apples, hopscotch. Go on, I know you're dying to!

Chapter 5

Dream Big: How to Get Anything You Want

Call me a dreamer, a hopeless romantic, even an optimistic crazy pants, but I believe you can manifest whatever you want in life. This book is living proof of it. The truth is that I always knew one day I would write a book. It felt inevitable, and at the beginning of 2012 I woke up with the feeling that it was time to start writing. It sounded great in theory, but the reality was a little more tricky. Let's run down the checklist:

- ♥ Great book ideas? *Obviously stacks of them!*

- ♥ Contacts? *Er none.*

- ♥ Literary agent? *A what?*

- ♥ Funding? *Not so much.*

- ♥ Any clue at all about how to publish a book?
  None whatsoever.

Clueless clearly needed guidance. I turned to a dear friend of mine. *Howdy Mr. Google. How do I publish a book?* It turned out it's quite complicated. *Go figure!* Apparently I needed an agent, contract, submission guidelines, and so on and so forth. Talk about a dream dampener. So I decided to do what any sensible person would, play pretend and imagine it would be a walk in the park. The plan of action: get creative, start typing, believing and visualizing, and deal with each road bump as it came. You may think that was a little naively optimistic, but four weeks into writing I opened up my inbox to an e-mail that read: 'Dear Christy, I hope you don't mind me contacting you out of the blue. I am the Editorial Director of Hay House and would like to commission you to write a book.' Now, I'm a big believer in the power of the mind, but that one made my jaw drop, especially since I hadn't even shared my grand plans. So here we are. Need proof this stuff works? Well, you're holding it right now.

Hot, healthy, happy magnet

Believe in your mind, because your beliefs shape your destiny. Our world is made from consciousness. Every teeny tiny thought sends waves out into the incredible web linking everything together. Want to know the magical secret to how this universe rolls? It's called the 'law of attraction,' meaning like attracts like. You, hot stuff, are a little magnet, pulling toward you whatever you hold in your consciousness. You believe it, feel it, think it, and *poof,* that energy comes to you. Your circumstances, relationships, and events are mirrored by your thoughts, feelings, and emotions. This is why living in wave response with those delicious feelings of connection, calm, happiness, and positivity brings a life that mirrors those positive emotions. Dumping stress is therefore key to helping you create a life with oodles of happiness.

When you're calm and relaxed this hooks you into your higher self and means you can hear the intuitive messages being broadcast over the loudspeaker system. The thoughts and emotions you send out into the world become part of the collective subconscious. Lodged into other people's subconscious, those with the knowledge, connections, and resources are attracted to help you. Want it in a nutshell? Always focus on what you want, not what you don't want.

Universal sorcery

The great news is that almost anyone can be hot, healthy, happy, because, as you now know, we are rarely trapped by bad genes. No matter where you are in your life, you can change things. It all begins by working in cahoots with your subconscious, because she is the gatekeeper to the universal sorcery. Visualizing what you want, what makes you happy, means she'll start sending out those positive messages.

What's more, your subconscious is totally gullible. You could April-fool her every day of the week and she would keep falling for the same joke. Since your brain has the power to visualize anything you want, you can have some incredible fun with your subconscious. Visualize scenes and dream scenarios over and over again, and she actually thinks these are real memories. The reason this is so great is because if your subconscious thinks you've already achieved something, she will start to bring you the resources you need. Obviously this can backfire if your conscious mind is rerunning worst-case scenarios. So you need to back talk your conscious mind and coax her round with promises.

So before you can positively change your life you need to wave goodbye to those not-so-hot memories and beliefs holding you hostage in the past. Think, ponder, explore. Why is this keeping you stuck? You'd hoped after a time it would lose its power, but your conscious mind keeps recharging it with mental energy. Replaying old scenes over and over again. With each replay, feelings of dread surge to the surface. Your subconscious thinks: *Hey, she wants more depressing stuff in her life.* You're virtually bellowing at your subconscious: 'Look at what happens to me. I am such a bad-luck magnet!' Her response: 'Well if you say so honey, here you go.' Bad images, past failures, heartache, sadness, deceit, abuse, worry, and anxiety come running as though your life depended on it. Your biography is not your destiny. Ditch the past pains, spring-clean your consciousness, box up the old and tired mental clutter, and make space for some new inspiration.

- -

☼ *Hot, Healthy, Happy: Coax your mind round*

Start by back talking to your conscious mind and coaxing her round with a few promises of how things could be; how you want them to be. Switch on that creative artist gene, grab an imaginary paintbrush and swirl up some beautiful, motivating, joyful imagery, beliefs, and emotions. Go for anything so exciting, so awe-inspiring you want to cartwheel down the road naked. Your subconscious will roll up her sleeves and get busy. Before you know it, the resources you require will be conjured up, along with those 'life really is incredible' experiences you crave.

- -

What if, though, no matter what you try, your life is on the disaster repeat cycle? You just keep facing the same junk over and over and over again. You manage to ditch one loser, only to fall head over heels for another cut from the same cloth. You yo-yo diet your way from celery to pastries and back to celery again. Many of us never tire of rinsing and repeating the same old stuff over and over and over again. We make promises and heartfelt pleas with all the gusto we can muster, but end up right back at the starting line before we realize what has happened. You can beat down that inner nag of yours a gazillion times, pep talk yourself to oblivion, and dream your way from Z-list to A-list, but if you don't get your subconscious mind on board you are going to be rinse and repeating till the curtain closes. It's time to bring out the big guns, lady. You need to dust off those negotiating skills and get down deep into the pandemonium of your subconscious mind.

⟨💡⟩ Schmoozing a stubborn subconscious

If you want to stop the rinse-and-repeat cycle then try this four-step plan for getting your subconscious mind on the hot, healthy, happy program.

1. Eat some humble pie

That's right, don't assume you know it all. Really listen to what your subconscious mind has to say. She is a treasure trove of wisdom on your specialist topic – you! Respect what she has to say. So put on your best reporter smile, pull out your bejeweled microphone and interview your subconscious. Here are some topics to converse about:

★ What am I afraid of?

★ What is holding me back from change?

★ Why do I keep sabotaging myself?

★ What is the positive intention behind this action?

Get down to what really matters. Don't let her off the hook. Quiz her for specifics. Real details. But always lavish her with praise, instead of judging what she sends your way.

2. Acknowledge the fear

'I hear what you are telling me and I am listening.' For example, maybe you consistently sabotage yourself every time you try to become healthier. Maybe the fear is actually a belief that losing weight means sacrifice and being unhappy. Honor this fear. Promise that if this happens you'll take action to change the method. Respect what is truly important and what you really want from your life. Thank that part of you that's been resisting up until now and explain you no longer need it.

continued on p.144

continued from p.143

3. Convince her you can do it!

Find success stories, testimonials, and positive examples of what you want to manifest in your life, because your subconscious will do what she believes is possible. Prove it will work. Make her certain.

4. Affirm the belief with a wisdom nugget

Create a positive belief around what you want to achieve. For example: 'I deserve good food, and eating this way makes me feel happy and healthy.' Rinse and repeat your wisdom nuggets instead of past pains and negative beliefs. Whisper them to yourself as you fall into dreamland, as you rouse from slumber, and during meditation.

Magical manifestation

So you've got down in the trenches with your subconscious and wrestled your fears, but identifying the source of your junk isn't enough to get you to the finish line. You need some transformation-a-go-go to get you over the final hurdle. So how about if you let it all go and changed? Right now. What would life be like if your past wasn't holding you captive. Imagine you have a fairy godmother who, with a wave of her wand, declares: 'From now on you can be whatever and whoever you want. Let's just forget the times you messed up, those days you were a bit gossipy and a little unkind, all the heart-wrenching and incredible ways you have tried to feel loved. Let's start afresh, and while we're at it, let's forget the bruises, heartache, abuse, and neglect you faced along the way.'

What if you just forgot the past? Free spirit? Nothing to hang on to? Nothing left to despair about or resent? Fresh new you? Now a-go-go. Who would you want to be? Get your thinking cap on because it's time for my visualization master class. Buckle up your seatbelt and keep your arms in the vehicle at all times, because it's going to be a whirlwind ride. Need some last-minute inspiration? Well here are some of the things that I have manifested in my own life:

- ♥ I created a kickass business.
- ♥ I got my first TV job.
- ♥ I overcame my sucky ill health.
- ♥ I found my gorgeous hunky husband.
- ♥ I now have a crazy and enchanting little girl.
- ♥ I published my first book.
- ♥ Lots of little things too naughty and delicious to share here... sorry!

Your imagination is your limit. I believe you can use the power of creative visualization for whatever you want to achieve or manifest in your life. You'll never really know till you try. Obviously, flying and becoming invisible would be cool, but perhaps start with things you believe are conceivable. Learn to walk before you can fly, so to speak! Visualization is a key ingredient to hot, healthy, happy. It has been integral to my success, so see what you can hustle up.

⠠⃝ Visualization 101

Here is my guide to visualizing successfully. You don't need to be a Harvard graduate to get this right; after all you've been daydreaming all your life (*I hope!*). But if you want to supercharge your results then learning a few techniques might really help.

Step 1: Write a dream plan
It is likely when you start that you'll experience crazy thoughts, hurtling wildly between your ears at a million miles an hour. So start by writing yourself a dream plan to keep yourself on track. Focus

continued on p.146

continued from p.145

on how you want to feel. For example, if you want to run your own business, start by thinking how that would feel:

★ It feels awesome to be my own boss and make my own decisions.

★ I feel proud of myself for creating a successful and meaningful business.

★ I feel incredibly confident, and destined for ongoing success.

So take action now. Write down some key points on what you want to focus on. Now let's move on.

Step 2. Relax and turn up the inner peace

Throw a 'Do Not Disturb' sign on the door, take the phone off the hook and make yourself comfy. Give yourself at least five minutes or so of downtime before whipping up those visualizations. Follow the relaxation exercise for reconnecting with your inner child in the previous chapter (see pages 135–136).

Step 3: Start to visualize

Imagine yourself acting the way you would act if you'd already achieved your goals. The key is to make the pictures in your mind as vivid and dazzling as possible. Be the 'you' that you want to be. Look around and notice your surroundings. Where are you? Who else is there? Are they happy and in control like you? Chat with them. Notice how you look, feel, talk, and act as this confident, successful person. Make the images as detailed as possible. How do others respond to you? Look? Feel? Act? Notice what you are doing and how you are doing it. Pay attention to every little detail.

The more lifelike your visualizations, the better the results. You're planting new seeds in your consciousness compost. Make it more vivid and detailed than a real memory and you'll get better results. It's all about creating bright, attractive pictures in your mind. Remember to act how you want to be when visualizing, as if you already have it all at your fingertips. Focus on generating the same feelings you'd have if you had already achieved your goals: strong, intense emotions. Feel the success.

Another technique with magnetic pulling power is a vision board. All you need to do is find pictures of things you love and stick them on a pin board. *Ta dah!* But the trick to making the magic happen is to escape the cultural ideals of a perfect life *(cue images of stacks of cash, exotic beaches, the perfect partner, you name it)* and get frisky with that genetically unique angel within you who radiates your dreams and ideals. As you begin to collect pictures that resonate with your higher self, you unlock one of your incredible superpowers: your imagination. Crafting and creating images will glue certain events and objects into your subconscious mind, helping her steer your choices toward making the vision real.

☀ Create a vision board

How you create your vision board – on paper or on your computer desktop – is up to you, but this is my three-step plan for turning those images into something tangible that you can manifest in your life.

Step 1: Make your inner angel fly
Tell your conscious mind to take the night off and let your inner angel choose. Leaf through magazines, walk through the world (real or virtual), and go for anything that makes you gasp, salivate, sob, double take, or tingle.

You'll know you're on the right tracks when you feel it in your belly, heart, lungs, and big toe – any place that isn't your over-thinking brain. Forget making sense. Experience will prove to you that collating these pictures in one place will start sparking something past your conscious mind's ability. If you're not already hoarding images that make your heart sing, keep your eyes open. Wherever you see them, get grabby.

Step 2: Go with the flow, mentally and emotionally
Most people rock step 1 without a hiccup: rummaging and amassing mesmerizing images by the basket-load. This is where you need

continued on p.148

continued from p.147

to focus, or not, as the case may be. The next step involves doing something that is completely the opposite of what we've had drummed into us our whole lives: NOT THINK. Can you imagine, *'Okay boys and girls, today we are going to practice not thinking.'* *Revolutionary!* To do it, you need to relax completely and blank your mind. Concentrate on not concentrating. Don't let your conscious mind criticize, over-scrutinize, or bully your board. Your board needs healthy boundaries! Back off analytical mind and let it be. Now for the trickiest step of all...

Step 3: Take action

A vision board is not a one-way ticket to paradise; you also need some elbow grease, so when opportunities come knocking then pay attention and grab them with both hands. They might not appear exactly the way you had anticipated, but that doesn't mean these won't work out better in the long run. This is why it is more helpful to aim for feeling a certain way (e.g. feeling secure) instead of going after specific conditions (e.g. more money). Otherwise you risk reaching your goal but still feeling exactly the same way as before. As you begin to take action, whatever little step you take will be reinforced by the universal witchcraft. It's quite happy to create whatever you can't.

There you go. You're a visualizing mastermind. Whoa! Now go dream us up a double helping of something fabulous. When a hot, healthy woman is fuelled with passion, a mission, and a vision board, watch out world.

On a final note, no matter whether you do or don't take my word for any of this – *creating your reality out of consciousness!* *Bah humbug!* – just give it a go. Even if it's just for a laugh, for kicks, a pastime, a fun experiment on a rainy afternoon. Who knows, something amazing might just happen after all, and when it does I want to hear all about it!

Hot, Healthy, Happy action plan

♥ Your beliefs shape your destiny. Like attracts like. So focus on staying in wave response: happy, calm, and positive to attract more of the same into your life.

♥ Start working in cahoots with your subconscious. Coax her round and start convincing her that what you want is achievable.

♥ Say goodbye to the stinking thinking holding you back. Smash those old tapes haunting you with past negativity; box them up and let them go. Start replaying images of success and happiness on repeat.

♥ Become a visualizing mastermind and daydream your way to the life you want.

Part IV

Hot, Healthy, Happy Life: The HHH 21-day Diet

Chapter 1

Ingredients for a Hot, Healthy, Happy Life

You create your life. What you eat, drink, and think makes you who you are. It isn't written in your genes. It doesn't come from out there. It all happens inside you. You're the master dreamer. The CEO. The one who conjures up her existence each and every day: what you look like, what you see, what you feel, and what comes into your life is up to you. This isn't about blame; it's about taking back your power. Discovering that YOU HAVE A CHOICE. You can change, and have an awesome time in the process. In the following chapters I'm going to be walking you through the HHH 21-day diet one day at a time. First, I want to teach you the recipe to a hot, healthy, happy life.

CAUTION: *These ingredients may cause transformations.*

Ingredient 1: A miracle-maker mindset

You: hot, healthy, happy. Can you see it yet? Because this is where it starts. To create it you have to believe it, feel it, visualize it, and dream about it. Convince your subconscious mind it's possible. Declare your superpowers and show her your intentions. Paint it with your mind. The more you think it, live it, feel it, and practice it, the harder it will be to go back to the old ways. You rewire for a different you. Your neurochemistry and neural pathways begin to change, and slipping up doesn't feel so comfy anymore. It's like the soft spot on the sofa suddenly became too big for your slim *derrière*. Your thoughts carve a new road for your body and your life, and now they're all free-flowing like an avalanche in that direction. This is the miracle mindset.

Being a miracle-maker begins by following your bliss. You were born to be happy. The more relaxed and at peace you are, the happier you'll feel. Happiness and health are soul mates: made for one another. According to Candace Pert[1], we have bliss hardwired into our physiology. Eliminating toxins, trauma, stinking thinking, and toxic relationships is only half the story – we also need to add in nutrients, sunshine, hugs, starlight, big dreams, and all the things that make us weak at the knees with joy.

We need to wake up thrilled and excited about what is ahead of us each day. Less 'No' and more 'Oh, yes!' Less 'I'm fine' more 'Wow, I rock!' So take time to find out what you love. Discover what is so incredible that every day it makes you throw back the quilt and run down the stairs. Do whatever gives your life meaning and purpose. Whatever makes you shine. Follow your bliss unicorn, and you'll find life flows.

Ingredient 2: Going with the flow...

Say goodbye to stress and begin to take joy seriously. Laugh your head off. Let it boost your immune system, protect you from viruses, and soothe your stress levels. Prescribe yourself a daily dose of whatever or whoever gives you that sidesplitting belly laugh. A great chuckle is a daily essential. Remember, your brain mirrors the world around you. It mimics what you show it. Happiness, joy, laughter, downright craziness, we feel that stuff right to our core. We suck it up and resonate with it from every angle. So pick your people wisely. Get chummy with the happy, go-with-the-flow people living their dreams and send the doomers 'n' gloomers and drama queens to the answerphone. Stake your energy vampires and give your life force to the people and parts of your life that give you love back. Be a healthy boundary babe and live life on your terms.

Ingredient 3: Be an alkalizing angel

To be hot, healthy, happy you need to create an alkaline pH in your body. Alkaline means healthy, vibrant, radiant, and clear. Modern diets and lifestyles with high meat, grains, sugar, pollution, alcohol, tobacco, stimulants, and stress can have you low on the pH scale. They make your body acidic. Think acidic then think yeast, viruses, autoimmune conditions, and even cancer. If, like me, you were too busy eyeing up some hottie to pay attention in chemistry at school, you may need a quick recap on pH balance. The pH scale goes from 0–14, with 7 being neutral. Anything below 7 is acidic, and above 7 is alkaline. Ideally, our optimal blood level should be 7.365. This is important, because the pH of our internal fluids affects every cell in our body. You might say that chronic over-acidity is the root of all sickness... and it also keeps you overweight. *Now I have your attention!* The HHH 21-day diet will give your meals an alkaline makeover, so around 80 percent of your plate will be filled with alkaline foods and only 20 percent acid. Of course, 100 percent alkaline is awesome when the mood takes you. However, forget overwhelm and perfection. You don't need to be an acid and alkaline whiz kid. Think little shifts. To start, just lean into it and notice what happens.

Ingredient 4: Nourishment not stimulation

If you're living on the red line of biochemical debt, it's time for a stimulation shakedown. Surviving on refined sugars, stimulants, and caffeine is like splurging every day with a credit card. Red lippy, Mulberry bag, Kurt Geigers, swipe, swipe, swipe. Instant pleasure, but the bill is in the mail. We always pay later, and with interest, crashing more exhausted than when we started. Surviving on stimulants to keep us going is simply flashing one credit card to pay another. As any shopaholic will attest this is a disaster waiting to happen. If you want to be hot, healthy, happy you need to get back in touch with your natural energy and it comes from nourishment. Forget Band-Aiding fatigue and irritability with stimulation. Clear your biochemical debt and start making investments in your energy, health, and looks.

The HHH 21-day diet is packed with nutrient-dense whole foods that will get you clear of the red line. Every day, make big nutrient investments and eliminate the need for stimulation. Keep your blood sugar level steady with good quality protein, low-GL carbohydrates, and good quality fats. Don't allow yourself to be sabotaged by the four energy robbers: caffeine, sugar, alcohol, and nicotine. Before you eat, drink, or invest energy thinking about something, ask yourself: will this be nourishing or stimulating? If it's the latter then say goodbye, let it go. Little word of encouragement: your brain may have a screaming match with you for a few days as you come off stimulants, and headaches, feeling tired, sugar cravings, and irritability are par for the course. Keep adding in the nourishment and stay strong – it will be worth it, I promise!

Ingredient 5: Getting more for less

Now I don't know about you but I love a bargain; I love things that are simple: little work with huge rewards, small loss for big gains. Eating is no different. I want maximum nutrients to make me look and feel great with the least amount of effort possible. That's why nutrient-dense whole foods are a no-brainer: maximum goodness, minimal work. Supercharged with little digestive energy. Nowadays most of us are overfed and undernourished. Puffy and swollen, yet exhausted and depleted. This is because most of what we eat is devoid of vitality. Food processed within an inch of its life, bulked up with fillers, preservatives, sweeteners, and flavors. These foodstuffs lack essential nutrients and are hard work for the body to break down. They leave you lacking.

Have you ever been friends with an energy vampire? You know, the drama queen who literally sucks the energy from your life, giving you little in return. Processed foods demand energy and nutrients. They take, take, take without loving you back. Your body's job is to convert the energy from your chow into energy that it can use. It's not a straight swap: to do this you use up energy. The more processed junk you eat, the more energy it needs to use. Anti-nutrients in these foodstuffs also use up sexy nutrients just to process them. For example, a jar of pasta sauce could be packed with sweeteners, fillers, and preservatives. You may not notice them but your body does. It needs to use up nutrients to process these. Instead, spend a few extra minutes making your own. Simple, fresh ingredients are a clear winner. They give instead of taking. Be smart. Get more for your time and effort. Eat foods that give back, give you energy, vitality, glow and shine. You're worth it.

Ingredient 6: Going allergen free

Many of us live with persistent, unexplained symptoms; we just never feel 100 percent right. Often it's our ongoing diet that's behind these symptoms. The most common mood reactions are anger, irritability, stress, depression, and hyperactivity. Physical reactions can be respiratory, asthma, sore throat, earache, and stuffy nose. Digestive problems appear as constipation, bloating, stomach pain, gas, reflux, and heartburn. Unlike an allergic reaction, intolerances don't necessarily rear their ugly heads straight after eating the offending food. They can appear days or even a week later. Common food intolerances include:

- Gluten (e.g. wheat, and often barley, rye, and oats)

- Dairy milk products

- Soya, nightshades (e.g. tomatoes, peppers, white potatoes, aubergine/eggplant, and tobacco)

- Chocolate, peanuts, and high salicylate foods (e.g. apples and oranges)

- Shellfish

To be hot, healthy, happy you need to remove the foods that cause a reaction. Try eliminating gluten and dairy first. See what happens. There is little chance of you being able to find any processed refined foods in the grocery store that won't contain at least one common allergen. Corn and soya are particularly problematic. Cheap and stable they are the perfect set of ingredients for filling out processed foods. Nightshades (tomatoes, peppers, etc.) have been associated with pain conditions, so if you have fibromyalgia, chronic back pain, joint pains, etc. then try excluding these during the 21 days, too.

Ingredient 7: Raw foods

To be hot, healthy, happy harness the power of raw foods. Leafy greens, veggies, wheatgrass, spirulina, sprouts, low-GL fruits, nuts, seeds, gluten-free grains, seaweed, vegetable juices, and smoothies will fill your system with chlorophyll, vitamins, minerals, phytonutrients, fiber, enzymes, and oxygen. Hot, healthy, happy cells are in love with oxygen. They stay gorgeous with an alkaline, oxygen-rich, high-plant-based diet. Those nasty villains – yeasts, bacteria, and pathogenic bacteria – love an acidic diet high in animal products, processed foods, refined sugars, stimulants, and synthetic chemicals. A high-raw-plant-based diet helps your body cruise the alkaline waves. More oxygen means healthier cells. Raw and living foods are the greatest alkaline oxygen-rich foods you can eat. They're the ultimate ingredients of the HHH 21-day diet. Not only will you get a greater amount of nutrients, they will also help you lose weight.[2,3] You don't need to be 100 percent raw (although it also makes food preparation easier), because this program is not about absolutes. But upping your intake of raw foods and removing the processed, denatured foods is a big step in the right direction.

☼ Hot, Healthy, Happy: Ravish raw foods

Raw foods contain delicious life force. So include lots with each of your meals. Lightly steam or gently steam-fry foods, keeping them below 150°C (300°F) Gas Mark 2. Over this temperature, essential fatty acids turn to trans fats. *Hello inflammation.* Avoid charred and BBQ foods at all costs, and if roasting then slow roast in the oven with plenty of liquid or oil, and keep turning the veggies (or whatever you're cooking) to avoid charring.

Ingredient 8: A green juice a day

Are you ready to discover the ultimate healthy fast food? Raw green vegetable juices and green smoothies. *Yes, that's right, hot stuff.* Alkalizing, nutrient-packed, energy dense, easy to digest, chlorophyll and oxygen rich, raw, and low GL. Whoa! They really are the perfect food. If you're ready to say goodbye to poor health and embrace the gorgeous new you, then grab the juicer and smoothie machine from the back of the cupboard, dust them off and get busy. Don't be put off by the look of these concoctions. I admit green smoothies do resemble lawn mower pulp, but they're scrumptious. Not only that, drinking veggie juices and smoothies literally floods your system with alkalizing nutrients, giving your whole system a surge of enzymes, oxygen, and vitamins straight into your bloodstream. Although fruit-based smoothies may be tasty, they can also be very high in sugar. I always aim to make my smoothies and juices low glycemic load, so they are high in green leafy vegetables with only a little fruit to sweeten them (see pages 243–245). Packed with chlorophyll, that glass of green juice really is like having a big glass of sunshine!

- -

☼ Hot, Healthy, Happy: Go green

Start every day with about 570ml–1.2L (1–2 pints) of green juice or a green smoothie. These are incredible for curbing sugar cravings. If at night you can feel your fingers twitching for munchies just get that juicer out again and give your body another hit.

- -

Ingredient 9: Plant protein

Vegetarian, paleo, pescatarian, or vegan? *Oh the controversy.* The way I see it, animal flesh is only as healthy as the animal it came from. Before you chomp down on that steak or chicken breast consider how the animal lived. If you choose to eat meat, opt for free-range organic, as the animal will have had less exposure to chemicals and antibiotics. The HHH 21-day diet doesn't include red meat, game or poultry, so that should reduce your exposure to hormones, antibiotics and pesticides as much as possible, but for ease I've kept in fish and eggs. These should not be the star of the show, but may make it easier for you to cut out dairy and wheat. We live in a polluted world so go for wild deep-sea fish and always opt for organic free-range eggs.

☼ *Hot, Healthy, Happy: Food combining*

Proper food combining is also crucial on the HHH 21-day diet. Animal products are acidic, so eat them with lots of leafy greens and non-starchy vegetables (preferably raw). Teaming them with starchy carbohydrates (e.g. potatoes, pasta, noodles, or rice) will only slow down your digestive system.

Eating meat is a personal choice, but quality is paramount. Be picky. Don't just throw the faceless plastic packet into your shopping basket, be an informed and empowered individual. Animal protein doesn't need to be center stage. The HHH 21-day diet favors plant-based proteins like quinoa, amaranth, spirulina, buckwheat, millet, and hemp products. There are also many incomplete plant-based proteins such as seeds, nuts, lentils, and pulses. Don't take incomplete to mean inferior, especially when you are eating a fabulous varied diet like the HHH.

ᗺ Junk food vegetarian alert

I've seen many people grow a conscience, turn vegetarian, and pack their diet (not to mention their rear ends) with pasta, dairy, mock meats, and processed soya. Substituting fish and meat for mock meats, soya, and dairy is not the path to a healthy life. Soya has become the fast-food option of the vegetarian world; it's the processed, packaged, throw-in-the-oven alternative to meat. Mock meats, veggie mince, mock chicken, mock fish, soya milk, soya cheese – the list is endless. Processed, processed, and processed some more. I like to call this fat vegetarian syndrome. I imagine you can think of a few people in your life suffering from this condition. Not a good look. Needless to say, these foods don't belong on this program.

Ingredient 10: Raw plant fats

Are you a fat phobe? Then the HHH 21-day diet will be your fat rehab. Fat is not the enemy. On the contrary, it is absolutely essential if you want to be slim and healthy. But before you start downing the oil in a bid to get hot, you need to remember that, just like the wrong kind of sugar, the wrong kind of fat does damage. What many people don't realize is that the wrong fats create a greater need for fat than the body requires. In other words, if you consistently put in the bad, damaged fats then the body will continue to crave the good fat it really needs. So eat fat, but be selective.

Raw plant fats are awesome: avocados, cold-pressed oils, seeds, and nuts are packed with essential fatty acids such as omega-3 and omega-6. Like the essential amino acids, we can't make them so we need to get them from our food. The list of health benefits of these omega warriors is endless. Keep cravings at bay and extinguish the need for willpower by having an oil change. Take out the processed, packaged foods. Say goodbye to soya, canola, corn oils, hydrogenated vegetable oil, and margarine spreads that all contain trans fatty acids. Add in raw plant fats and just a little dairy butter for cooking. Now we're talking!

Here are some of the delicious fats to enjoy:

- ♥ Cold-pressed oils

- ♥ Avocados

- ♥ Raw nuts and nut butters – nuts are very dense foods and should only be consumed in moderation. If you feel your system is quite toxic then I would keep nuts to a minimum until you feel it is ready.

- ♥ Raw coconut and coconut butter.

- ♥ Seeds: pumpkin, sunflower, chia, hemp, flax, and sesame.

♥ EPA and DHA can be found in oily fish such as salmon, mackerel, and herring, but avoid tinned varieties and shellfish. If you prefer to avoid fish, then try some algae.

Ingredient 11: Hydrate, hydrate, hydrate

You know that thick, heavy feeling in your head, the dull headache, that sudden anxious feeling from nowhere, the restlessness at night when you're trying to drift off, and even that swelling in your ankles? *What do we call those? Oh yeah, kankles!* These are all signs that you need some liquid loveliness. Drinking filtered water is like showering down your insides. Trading your diet drinks for water is an act of liberation.

Our bodies are around 60–70 percent water and our brain is around 80 percent *(and you thought it was just air and dust in there)*. The delicious H_2O escorts those sexy nutrients into your cells while washing the acid wastes out. Respiration, urine, and sweat mean we lose up to 1.7L (3 pints) of water a day, and this needs to be replenished. When you're having fresh vegetable juices, herbal teas, salads, and raw veggies these all count toward your daily requirement. Keeping yourself hydrated is the key to stopping yourself from overeating. Your body says, 'I'm thirsty' and your brain says, 'Right, where did I put that box of cookies?' So stay hydrated and keep those cravings under control. It's a win–win situation.

Just to be clear, flavored water, coffee, fizzy juice, black tea, bottled juice, and energy drinks are not water. Yes, even vitamin water! If it has sugar or artificial sweeteners then leave it alone. You aren't quenching your thirst, so stop protesting and just remove them from your drinking repertoire. You can overdose on water, too; moderation is key in life and this is no different. Use your brain: it's not rocket science. Stay hydrated by drinking regularly and keep it moderate: aim for 6–8 glasses of water in a day. Sometimes less is more.

☼ How clean is your water?

Let's talk about the plastic water bottle. Most bottled waters are acidic and costly, and the plastic lasts for thousands of years! Our poor planet. For the sake of your health, and our whales and wildlife, stop buying them. A good option is an under-sink filter, such as a reverse osmosis filter. This allows you to not only drink this clean water but also wash and cook your food in it. If this is out of your budget, at least invest in a filter jug. You can go another step further and use a whole-house water system. Again, if this is too pricey, then buy a cheap shower filter head and add a chlorine ball to your bath. Run your bath with the windows open and then give it ten minutes or so before stepping in. This should help reduce your exposure to chlorine.

Ingredient 12: Detox your environment

There's no doubt we live in a toxic world, surrounded by potentially harmful substances. Everyday products resemble science experiments loaded with hundreds of dangerous synthetic chemicals. It's time to become a natural beauty. Don't worry, I'm not suggesting a make-up fast, just a lotions and potions upgrade. Nowadays there are some incredible non-toxic beauty products available. Ideally you want to avoid those with synthetic fragrance and instead go for ones labeled 'no added fragrance' or 'natural fragrance'. With so many delicious essential oils available there is no need for synthetics anyway. Next you want to avoid the estrogen mimics. Pick products without parabens (e.g. methylparaben, butylparaben, etc.). Check out www.thefoodpsychologist.com for all the products I love.

Now it's time to check out the household cleaning products. Aim to dump any heavy-duty stuff and replace it with natural alternatives (environment-friendly brands are also human friendly). As much as possible, avoid using pesticides or herbicides on your plants, and reduce your reliance on over-the-counter drugs. Buy organic foods where possible, and peel non-organic fruits and veg. Before storing, wash and soak your fresh produce in water and vinegar to remove any pesticide residue and wax. Restrict your exposure to plastics by removing foods from plastic packaging before storing. Cook with stainless steel pots and pans. These are just a few simple changes you can make to reduce your exposure, and they will positively benefit your health.

Ingredient 13: Glow

Over the years I have discovered a few little tricks that, when practiced repeatedly, will have your skin soft, glowing, and gorgeous:

Body brushing

Dry skin brushing shifts dead skin cells, stimulates acupressure points, gets your lymphatic system dancing and your circulation singing, and is fabulous for eliminating cellulite. If you're prone to scaly, dry patches and ingrown hairs, then get ready for a new you. You can pick up a natural bristle brush from your local pharmacy. Use on dry skin, ideally just before you step into the shower or bath. Be gentle. For those cellulite-prone areas, use circular motions. Glide from your feet up your body, over your tummy, and up your arms, always working toward your heart. Brush every day and wash the brush once a week with soap and let it dry.

- -

☼ Hot, Healthy, Happy: Have some cider in the bath

If you suffer from vaginal infections, yeast or urinary infections, add 240–480ml (8–16fl oz) of apple cider vinegar to your bath to help restore a good balance. Antibiotics, poor hygiene, and a high-sugar diet can leave your lady bits a little yeasty! Grab the apple cider vinegar and hit the bath. This is also great for joint pain, arthritis, and gout.

Epsom salts and baking soda baths

These can help your body eliminate acid wastes from your cells and tissues. You only need add 225–450g (8–14oz) of Epsom salts and 50g (2oz) of baking soda to your bath and you're good to go. The sulphate in the Epsom salts is absorbed through the skin and can soothe the digestive tract, while magnesium helps your muscles relax and can aid sleep. These baths can also be beneficial for removing heavy metals and radiation, reducing inflammation, and soothing skin conditions such as psoriasis and eczema.

CAUTION: *If you're suffering from diabetes, high blood pressure, or kidney disease, or are pregnant or breastfeeding, avoid or limit the use of Epsom salts as you may have an increased chance of adverse effects.[4] Always consult your medical practitioner before using Epsom salts if you suffer from a medical condition, or are taking medication.*

Infrared saunas

I talk about infrared saunas in Part II (see page 87), but they are so amazing I just want to shout their praises again. They give you the ultimate glow, clear your skin, and are unsurpassed for shifting the build-up of heavy metals, plastics, and environmental toxins from your cell tissues. I have a one-person infrared sauna which just plugs into the wall. It is by far the best way to relax in the evening. Facing a skin detox breakout? This clears it. Those with fatigue and pain conditions will also benefit from its healing powers. You can buy these as foldaway tents where your head sticks out, or as wooden saunas.

Ingredient 14: Shaking that booty

You want to know what the best exercise in the world is? Whichever one you love. That's right, do what works for you. To be hot, healthy, happy our body needs around 30–35 minutes of heart-pumping exercise five times a week. This isn't a big commitment. Throw on those sweatpants and a hoodie and get shaking and shifting. Weight-bearing exercises are awesome: kinky kettle bells, and dazzling dumbbells. Bounce bonanza on your rebounder first thing. Hula-hoop, Zumba, hit the streets for a power walk, hike or bike through the mountains. Let your lungs flood with oxygen while you soak up the fresh air and sunshine.

- -

☼ Hot, Healthy, Happy: Bounce baby

I love rebounding: it massages and stimulates the lymph system, helping the body eliminate and increase oxygen. It's also fantastic for digestion and is gentle on the joints. Start with 15 minutes in the morning and work up to 30 minutes five times a week.

- -

Ingredient 15: Beauty sleep

Losing vital beauty sleep is treacherous for your health and wellbeing. Hitting the sack early and getting to sleep by 11 p.m. could solve many of your day-to-day symptoms. Headaches, sugar cravings, moodiness, and fatigue are all signs that you're lacking in the sleep department. Ideally, aim to finish your last meal about three hours before your head hits the pillow. This way your body can turn its energy toward cleansing. If you eat too late, your body will need to use this precious repair and rejuvenation time to break down your food. Instead it should work away while you're in peaceful slumber, repairing muscles, your memory, your hormones, and your metabolism. If you live like a night owl, chances are you're hitting the refrigerator for midnight snacks. Hit the hay earlier and save that waistline.

Routine is key for healthy sleep, so establishing a good habit of going to bed and waking up at the same time is great practice. Stress, shift work, and modern living affect the body's ability to self-wake. We can't catch up on sleep, so over doing it at the weekend can just throw you out of sync. Give yourself a stimulant shakedown and keep away from caffeine, depressants, alcohol, and strenuous exercise a few hours before sleep time.

- -

☼ Hot, Healthy, Happy: Enjoy some down time

When life gets crazy, take a nap. If you have a dip between 1 p.m. and 3 p.m. maybe you need some more rest. Recharge. Give yourself a power nap for 20 minutes, hiding out somewhere comfy. Set your phone timer and off you go. *Zzzzzzzz*

- -

Ingredient 16: Sunshine

Bring more sunshine into your life. Boost your immune system, make more happy chemicals, recharge your energy, strengthen your nerves, heal your dry skin, and dose your system with vitamin D. If you're a porcelain-skinned honey like me, you may be hiding in the shadows like one of the characters from *Twilight*. After all, sun equals FRECKLES, MOLES, SUN DAMAGE, and CANCER. *Nasty.* The only time you step into light is when you're slathered head to toe in sun cream. But really, why would the very thing that energizes us, keeps us alive, makes us glow, also make us sick and kill us? Mr. Sunshine Scapegoat: it's not the sun, we do that to ourselves.

It's all about what we put on and in the body that makes us sick. Toxic sunscreens are packed with chemicals. We slather that junk all over us, then go outside and bake it into our skin. We make our bodies weak and sun sensitive by feeding ourselves garbage. If our system is over-toxic and our kidneys overworked, then the body shoves all that nasty stuff through our skin. Then the toxins sit there cooking on our skin in the sun.

But don't worry, there are plenty of good quality, natural, non-toxic sun creams available. Potions upgrade time. You can also feed your body nature's sunscreens from the plant kingdom: watermelon, oranges, carrots, blueberries, apricots, and leafy greens. Don't be afraid of the sun; instead, just be wise about it. Half-an-hour of glorious sun on a bright day (depending on where you live) will top up your vitamin D levels, so clean your body and then get out and bask in its glory. If you live where the sun never shines, or you're prone to the winter blues, then invest in a lightbox (see page 41). One hour every morning and you'll be shining bright and sleeping sound. Finally, gulp down your green juice and you'll slurp up the sun. Beautiful greens trap the sun's energy in chlorophyll. That big glass of green juice really is sunshine in a glass. *Delicious and frisky fresh.*

Ingredient 17: Daily meditation

Meditation is vital for hot, healthy, happy. When you feel strong and centered, emotional negative thinking and turmoil don't have the same sabotaging effects. Meditation is perfect first thing in the morning and is ideal for setting you up for the day. However, unless you're a Zen meditation master, the thought of meditation may feel overwhelming. Your mind resembles a rave party – wild, untamed, and busy. Jumping around. I can relate. But a chaotic mind means a chaotic body, so let's create a spiritual rave by getting in touch with the meditation pillow and quieten the chaos and chatter. Calming the conscious mind allows us to connect with our higher self and is one of the perks of meditation.

A peaceful mind equals a peaceful body. Start with five minutes in the morning and the same in the evening. Then work up to 20 minutes. Give yourself some calm space for your mind to rest.

Here's the great news: anyone can meditate. It doesn't matter if you've never met a monk or you think the Dalai Lama might be related to Dolce & Gabbana, you can still learn to be still. All you need is a comfortable place to sit or lie and a blanket to keep your tootsies toasty. Allow your body to be peaceful and simply focus on your breath. If your mind begins to run riot, just return your focus to your inward and outward breaths. Think of your mind as being like a wild, untamed horse. It's going to run wild. Just accept it. Sure, you can watch it galloping around like crazy. Just don't jump on its back and ride off! Instead observe the thoughts and one by one, breathe them away.

☼ Hot, Healthy, Happy: Guided meditation

If you're new to meditation and struggling to quieten the internal chatter, consider investing in some meditation CDs to take you through the steps. Chanting music can also help to calm your conscious mind.

So now you know the secret ingredients to a hot, healthy, happy life, let's start putting them into action...

Chapter 2
Getting Started

Ready to take the plunge? Awesome, then let's get down to business. Over the next 21 days you'll be changing your brand. Every day you'll be making big investments in how you look and feel by focusing on the way you eat, drink, and think. You're going to live with purpose and strive for the body and life you want. Here's my five-step plan

1. Dump it.

2. Shop like a superstar.

3. Transition.

4. HHH 21-day diet.

5. Living hot, healthy, happy ever after.

Dump it

Start by throwing out whatever is keeping you stuck. Recruit your kitchen on your team. Make your cupboards and refrigerator hot, healthy, happy first, then your body will follow. When my fridge and kitchen cupboards are packed with delicious edibles, eating healthily becomes irresistible. However, if the inside of my fridge resembles a cake factory, a moment of hunger turns to self-sabotage faster than I can say double chocolate brownie. My brain can't resist. Set yourself up to succeed. Make your kitchen an eating sanctuary packed to the gunnels with fresh and easy to prepare whole foods. That way it's easier to make better choices. Make this a family affair and get everyone in the house on the hot, healthy, happy bus.

Below you will find my dump-it list. It might seem like a waste, but think about it this way. Wouldn't you rather waste the food than waste your chances of slim thighs, a calm digestive system, and an energetic body? Of course you would! Plus, you could donate any non-perishable items to your local food bank or homeless feeding program.

Once you've made space for the new, don't leave room for bingeing and regret. Create a home that supports a hot, healthy, happy you. Trust me, you will be restocking. Starving isn't on the agenda.

Here's what you need to bid adieu to:

- ♥ Gluten products: pasta, bread, noodles, pastries, cakes, cookies, wheat, and bran cereals. Have a little cry if you need to (*I know I did!*), but once you realize how great you'll feel when these aren't clogging up your digestion they'll soon lose their appeal.

- ♥ Refined sugars and artificial sweeteners: read the labels – if it contains sugar, corn syrup, aspartame, sucralose, artificial flavorings, or colorings, it has to go.

- ♥ Drinks: flavored water, fizzy drinks, cordials, coffee, and black teas.

- ♥ Refined, processed products: bottled sauces, white rice, table salt, etc.

♥ Dairy, soya, and substitute meat products: cheese, milk, yogurts, and mock meats. I know it seems tough, but living dairy-free for just 21 days will cleanse and clear your system – your digestive system and skin will love you for it.

♥ Animal products: get rid of the hormone-filled, antibiotic-packed, non-organic animal meats and eggs. Also, dyed, smoked, or farmed fish, and yes, that includes tinned varieties.

Shop like a superstar

All finished? Then it's time for a restock. Start by writing a shopping list. Don't risk getting side-tracked or dazed and confused by special offers, neon colors, price drops, and the products screaming their so-called health benefits. Once you get in the grocery store keep this in mind: spend most of your time in the fresh produce section and stock up on fresh foods; from there take a quick skirt around the edges, dipping in for the odd product here and there. The middle section of most grocery stores is usually packed with processed junk. Most big chains now have a specialist aisle of allergy and gluten-free health foods. You may find one or two things here, but beware of the fraudsters dressed up as health foods. They lurk everywhere. Be smart and read the labels. Don't let them sneak home with you!

🔅 The black art of label reading

Forget carbs, calories, and multiplying fat grams. Just read the ingredients. It doesn't matter about the calorie or fat mumbo jumbo. You don't need the government recommended daily allowances to tell you what to put in your mouth. Just read the ingredients. If they're healthy, wholesome, and clean, then throw them in your

continued on p.174

continued from p.173

shopping basket. If it contains refined sugar, white or bleached flour, hydrogenated oils, animal products, and artificial or synthetic junk then don't eat it. Simple? Ignore the nonsense on the labels promising miraculous things. Don't trust it. It is BS. 'Wholesome,' 'Wholegrain,' 'Natural' 'Low Fat.' Why would you take advice from companies, organizations, and agencies that put colorings, preservatives, hydrogenated oils, chemical preservatives, artificial flavors, and sweeteners into your foods? Ignore them. Live your life. Get hot, healthy, happy.

Once you've restocked head for the checkout. Now a word of warning: if you have been living on packaged foods you may have a slight heart attack when the cashier announces the total. Restocking on healthy, fresh foods is expensive because spices, seasoning, oils, and long-term staples can cost. Once you have these though they'll last ages, so just don't freak out. Your weekly receipt will drop once you have the basic essentials. Keep in mind that the price at the checkout doesn't show you the real cost. I think about all the doctors' visits, time off sick, and social events I used to miss. Choosing cheap non-foodstuffs in a bid to save a bit of money each week cost me a lot more. Think about the money you normally spend on takeouts, alcohol, medicine, and time feeling unwell. Now that's really pricey?

Hot, healthy, happy shopping list

Here's a rundown of my favorite foods. Awesome healers and nutritional superstars, these are my best friends nowadays. Let me introduce you. You don't need everything mentioned below, just follow your heart and go with the foods that rock your boat. If you haven't tried some of these then there is no better time than the present. Be adventurous and dive in.

Veggies, herbs, and leafy greens

Plant power is the cornerstone of the HHH 21-day diet. They're the stars of hot, healthy, happy:

- Spinach
- Kale
- Cabbage
- Brussels sprouts
- Broccoli
- Cauliflower
- Red chard
- Green beans
- Peas
- Ginger root
- Red and white onions
- Garlic
- Carrots
- Leeks
- Beetroot
- Sweet potatoes
- Butternut squash
- Parsnips
- Turnips
- Aubergines (eggplant)
- Mushrooms

- Asparagus
- Courgettes (zucchini)
- Spring onions (scallions)
- Celeriac
- Avocado
- Cucumber
- Bell peppers
- Celery
- Tomatoes
- Sweet corn
- Coriander (cilantro)
- Fennel
- Basil
- Watercress
- Romaine lettuce and salad leaves
- Oregano
- Parsley
- Chili
- Olives
- Sprouts (lentil, sunflower, beetroot, bean, etc.)

There are no hard and fast rules. Be creative. Mix them with seasonings, experiment with stir-fries, salads, soups, stews, smoothies, and juices. A word of warning on those pesky white potatoes: they're a little naughty as they play with your blood sugar levels, so don't overdo them. The odd baked potato or using boiled potatoes to thicken soups is fine, just don't become Mrs. Potato Head.

Fruit

All the following fruits are low GL, so are much lower in sugar:

- ♥ Apples
- ♥ Pears
- ♥ Lemons
- ♥ Limes
- ♥ Grapefruit
- ♥ Kiwis
- ♥ Grapes (white and black)

- ♥ Melon (all varieties)
- ♥ Oranges
- ♥ Blueberries
- ♥ Strawberries
- ♥ Raspberries
- ♥ Cherries
- ♥ Apricots

Tropical fruits (e.g. bananas, pineapple, mangoes, etc.) and dried fruits (e.g. dates, cranberries, raisins, etc.) have a much higher sugar content than the fresh fruits listed above; they are fine, just watch your quantities. For example, one date or half a banana has the same effect on your blood sugar as a whole pack of berries. Also, fruit is loaded with vitamins and minerals but it is slightly acidic, so just take it easy. Keep your intake to around 2–3 portions a day: one apple, a pack of berries, and a pear is more than enough. Fruit is a great snack, but not a substitute for leafy greens!

Beans and legumes

There are loads of different beans and pulses to choose from, and they make a great alternative to meat or soya in chilies, casseroles, and in Asian and Oriental dishes. Some of the staples include:

- Chickpeas
- Lentils (all varieties)
- Aduki
- White
- Kidney
- Black
- Pinto
- Limos
- Flageolet

If you find beans difficult to digest (or that they cause flatulence), then you may need to increase your levels of beneficial bacteria with a probiotic before you can really enjoy them. Dried beans need to be soaked overnight in double the quantity of water; add a strip of Kombu seaweed to the water to aid digestion. Remove the water and rinse before using them. Canned varieties are easy to use and are a great alternative; just check the label and make sure they don't contain any preservatives. Ideally, you want those canned just in water with no added salt, sugar, or vinegar. Rinse them thoroughly before use.

Fish, eggs, and soya

If you want to eat fish choose fresh wild fish from sustainable sources. Just for starters, pick up some of the following:

- Wild Alaskan salmon
- Cod
- Haddock
- Sardines
- Herring
- Mackerel

Stay away from smoked, dyed, and canned fish. If you want to eat eggs then always go for free-range organic eggs. Avoid the mock meats that are highly processed and go for soy products close to their natural whole form:

- Soybean
- Edamame
- Tempeh
- Miso
- Tamari
- Tofu (stick to a portion or so a week)

Gluten-free grains, breads, pastas, noodles, and rice

Going gluten free doesn't mean you need to swear off all your favorites. Just change your brand and substitute any of the following:

- Quinoa
- Buckwheat
- Millet
- Amaranth
- Brown rice
- Wild rice
- Buckwheat or brown rice noodles
- Brown rice or quinoa pasta
- Gluten-free oats
- Quinoa, buckwheat, or millet flakes
- Corn tortillas
- Rice paper

Pick up some gluten-free granola as a treat, and try sunflower and rice or quinoa and buckwheat breads, buckwheat pizza bases, specialty gluten-free breads (e.g. ciabatta), buckwheat pancakes, gluten-free cake mixes, flax crackers, blue corn tortillas, brown rice cakes, raw breads, and raw bites. You'll find there is so much to choose from; just check out a good health food store as they're a treasure trove for gluten-free goodies.

Natural sweetness

My favorite alternatives to sugar are:

- Stevia
- Maple syrup
- Yacon syrup
- Honey
- Agave nectar
- Xylitol
- Coconut nectar

Stevia and yacon don't elevate your blood sugar levels, and stevia is perfect if you have a candida infection. You can buy it in liquid form or in packets. Other good substitutes include evaporated cane juice, brown rice syrup, barley malt syrup, turbinado sugar, raw sugar, beet sugar, date syrup, maple syrup, and blackstrap molasses (always buy 100 percent pure organic products). These guys all contain enzymes, calcium, iron, potassium, protein, B vitamins, magnesium, folic acid, chromium, and fiber.

Gluten-free flours

If you like to bake your own bread, there are stacks of gluten-free flours, including amaranth, clack bean, potato, oat, millet, buckwheat, chickpea, nut, and flaxseed meal.

Dairy alternatives

Removing dairy products from your diet isn't as hard as you might think. Most grocery stores now stock an extensive selection of dairy-free milks. Some of my favorites are:

- Rice
- Oat
- Almond
- Hemp
- Coconut
- Quinoa

You'll usually find these in the long-life milk section (those kept in the fridge have added sugars). You can even make your own milks in the blender (see recipes, page 247). Delicious.

Cold-pressed oils and fats

Cold-pressed oils such as hemp seed oil, pumpkin seed oil, 3/6/9 blends, and olive oil are all great drizzled over salads and lightly steamed veggies. Raw avocados, raw coconut, coconut butter, and coconut oil are also amazing additions. When cooking, use oils that can withstand high temperatures, otherwise they become high in free radicals. Olive oil can be used at a low heat, but grape seed and coconut are better for cooking at higher temperatures. Other oils such as hemp, pumpkin, and flaxseed should be kept cold.

Seasonings

Fresh herbs and seasoning are preferable, and listed under the fresh produce, but dried herbs are useful substitutes. I keep a stash of essentials that can transform most meals:

- Mixed herbs
- Celtic or Himalayan sea salt
- Wheat-free tamari
- Braggs amino acids
- Dulse flakes
- Ginger powder
- Ground garlic
- Ground coriander (cilantro)
- Oregano
- Parsley
- Dill
- Rosemary
- Turmeric
- Thyme
- Curry powder
- Garam masala
- Chinese five spice
- Cinnamon
- Nutmeg
- Mustard seeds

- ♥ Mint
- ♥ Vanilla bean and alcohol-free pure vanilla

- ♥ Parsley
- ♥ Yeast-free vegetable stock cubes

These seasonings, combined with some of the natural sweeteners, nut butters, and even fermented foods, make amazing sauces and dressings.

Nuts, seeds, and spreads

Again, there is plenty of choice, and a few seeds sprinkled on a salad or soup make a great addition. Choose from:

- ♥ Pumpkin
- ♥ Sunflower
- ♥ Chia
- ♥ Hemp
- ♥ Flax
- ♥ Sesame

- ♥ Almonds
- ♥ Walnuts
- ♥ Macadamias
- ♥ Hazelnuts
- ♥ Pecans
- ♥ Pine nuts

Flax and chia are gelatinous seeds that are fabulous at binding to bile and excreting toxins out of the body. If possible buy fresh raw nuts and store them in the fridge or freezer. Ideally these should be soaked for a couple of hours in water before eating. Alternatively, opt for the ready-bagged ones. Just watch out for any added salt, flavorings, sugar, etc.

For spreads try:

- ♥ Raw almond butter
- ♥ Cashew nut butter

- ♥ Tahini
- ♥ Hazelnut butter

Omega seed and hempseed butters are super healthy, although not quite as scrumptious as the nut butters. Most people have only ever tried peanut butter, but this often contains dangerous molds that give off toxins known as aflatoxins (yes, even the organic ones). If you love peanut butter then I'm sure you'll love the other nut butters, too. I think they taste even better. However, if you're struggling to lose weight, go easy on the nuts! Finally, a little dairy butter on a baked potato, or for cooking, is fine, but don't overdo it because the aim is to avoid animal products.

Fermented foods

For a healthy digestive system and a youthful complexion you need to stock up on fermented foods:

- ❤ Sauerkraut
- ❤ Kimchi
- ❤ Unpasteurized apple cider vinegar
- ❤ Tempeh
- ❤ Unpasteurized white miso
- ❤ Nutritional yeast

Sauerkraut and kimchi (available in Oriental grocery stores) are excellent for enhancing your levels of beneficial bacteria. Nutritional yeast makes foods a little cheesy tasting, but this is different from the yeast in bread so don't worry about it exacerbating candida. Just don't skip fermented foods because they sound weird; they are incredible for adding flavor, but more importantly, for conquering sugar cravings and calming your digestive system. These are vital ingredients in the HHH 21-day diet!

Seaweeds

You may eat seaweed when you hit the sushi bar, but there are so many other ways it can be enjoyed in a healthy way. Other seaweeds that are great for throwing into salads are:

- ❤ Dulse
- ❤ Hijiki
- ❤ Wakame
- ❤ Arame
- ❤ Nori

Seaweed is packed with minerals such as iodine, which is difficult to get from our everyday diet. Nori sheets make delicious cooked or raw wraps. If you have hung up your sombrero because those wheat-laden fajitas have you bloated and aching, then grab some nori sheets and roll them round your veggies, guacamole, and jalapenos. Go on, give them a go – they're awesome!

Drinks

Letting go of fizzy sodas, pasteurized fruit juices, cordials, coffee, black tea, and energy drinks doesn't mean you'll be stuck drinking plain old water forever. How about trying one or two of the following:

- ❤ Coconut water
- ❤ Herbal teas
- ❤ Yerba mate
- ❤ Green or white tea
- ❤ Chia
- ❤ Kombucha
- ❤ Fresh vegetable juices
- ❤ Smoothies
- ❤ Dairy-free milkshakes

Snacks

Of course, snacks are on the list! The great news is there are lots of yummy store-bought snacks that you can enjoy. It is simply about reading the labels and finding good companies you can trust. In our shop we have a whole section that is dedicated purely to snack bars and healthy fizzy drinks. I just make sure they have no added sugar or artificial sweeteners, but instead use natural sweeteners. Here are some great ones to look out for:

- Blue corn tortilla chips

- Seed and nut bars (make sure they use fruit and natural sweeteners, see page 179, and contain no nasty extras).

- Roast vegetable chips

- Rice cakes

- Instant miso soup

- Oatcakes

- Popcorn

- Raw chocolate or organic dark chocolate (with at least 70–85 percent dark cocoa solids)

- Coconut water

- Junk-free fizzy energy drinks

Superfoods and protein powders

There was a time when I thought protein powders were for muscle-bound gym junkies, but now I can't imagine my smoothies without them. Choose vegan over whey-based powders for maximum benefit. Hemp is rich in protein and essential fatty acids, making it ideal for increasing the protein content of smoothies and lowering their GL. Pea or sprouted brown rice protein are also good choices.

Another way to supercharge your smoothies is to throw in some maca, lucuma, raw cacao, and carob powders. Maca is awesome for calming you down during times of stress, and giving you energy when you're feeling flat. If you have ever suffered from adrenal fatigue then this is the one to throw into your morning smoothie. Cacao and carob are delicious and packed with antioxidants.

I also love green powders made from dehydrated cereal grasses. These shouldn't be used instead of juicing, but are a lovely addition. Two popular ones are wheatgrass and barley grass. Wheatgrass is incredibly alkalizing and excellent for promoting healthy blood. It can normalize the thyroid gland to stimulate your metabolism, help with digestion, and promote weight loss. Barley grass has 11 times more calcium than milk, seven times more vitamin C and bioflavonoids than orange juice, and five times more iron than spinach. If you're vegetarian it's a wonderful addition to your diet as it contains significant amounts of vitamin B12. Barley grass juice contains anti-viral activities and can neutralize heavy metals (e.g. mercury) present in the blood.

Along with the green powders you can also take algae powders. Top of my list are the following:

- ♥ Spirulina: one of the highest known protein sources on Earth, with around 70 percent complete protein; it even beats a chunk of steak (which only consists of 25 percent protein once cooked).

- ♥ Marine phytoplankton: this is not only a complete protein source, but also contains EPA and DHA and is one of the highest mineral and antioxidant foods.

- ♥ Wild blue-green algae: this is packed with nutrients and is a great source of beta-carotene, B vitamins, and chlorophyll.

- ♥ Chlorella: another complete protein, with all the B vitamins, vitamin C and E, and many minerals. It's great for removing heavy metals from the body and strengthening the immune system.

Visit me at www.thefoodpsychologist.com for more information on superfoods.

Supplements

Vitamins, minerals, enzymes, oxygen, and phytonutrients are the building blocks to being hot, healthy, happy. The best way to get these is from an organic, plant-based, whole food diet. However, you may choose to supercharge your efforts with a few key supplements. These are not a substitute for healthy eating, but could be an addition to your healthy eating plan.

In Part II we covered a number of specific supplements designed to address particular imbalances, so refer to that section for the key nutrients beneficial for certain imbalances. The following supplements are the suggested basic formula.

Multivitamins and minerals

Nutrients work synergistically, so it is important to use a comprehensive multivitamin and mineral supplement to give you a good basic supply. I often hear the argument that we shouldn't need supplements if we are eating a healthy diet. But the truth is many of us have digestive issues which mean our bodies find it difficult to get the maximum nutritional benefit from food. Some days we get busy, and we don't eat enough of the good stuff. Illness, food intolerances, medications, and stress are just a few of the factors that can increase our need for nutrients.

Vitamin D

Most of us spend way too much time indoors, but we're designed to get sunlight every day. Our lack of sunshine can result in vitamin D deficiency, which places us at risk of fatigue, pain, cramps, weight gain, restless sleep, headaches, and poor concentration. If you want to know if you're vitamin D deficient, you can take a vitamin D test (check out www.thefoodpsychologist.com). Your daily requirement differs depending on where you live, so check out your government's recommended daily amounts prior to supplementing. The best vegetable sources of vitamin D are fresh water algae, sea vegetables, edible weeds, and shitake mushrooms.

Omega-3 supplements

Your body needs essential fatty acids along with vitamins and minerals, so a daily omega-3 supplement is a good idea. You can get omega-3 from fish oil or from algae if you're vegan. Aim for around 1000mg (1g) of EPA a day, although too much can thin your blood, which may be problematic for you. This is not a substitute for natural omega-3 in your diet from oily fish, seeds, nuts, beans, and cold-pressed oils (e.g. flaxseed and hemp seed oil).

Digestive enzymes, hydrochloric acid, and pepsin

Cultured veggies, apple cider vinegar, and proper food combining, as discussed in the previous chapter, are excellent for helping your digestive system break down foods. For optimal absorption, consider taking digestive enzymes with your meals. This will help to keep your food quarantine in working order. There are numerous types to choose from, and some supplements include more than ten different enzymes. The key ingredients to look for are as follows: protease for digesting protein; amylase for digesting carbohydrates; lipase for digesting fats; and cellulose for insoluble fiber. I prefer supplements with HCL (hydrochloric acid) and pepsin included.

CAUTION: *HCL, pepsin, and digestive enzymes are not suitable for those suffering from gastritis or ulcers, or those on certain medications. Always check with your medical practitioner before introducing supplements.*

Probiotics and prebiotics

As discussed in Part II, we need good levels of beneficial bacteria (our doormen) to keep the digestive tract healthy. The truth is, there are lots of factors that can kill off the good guys, leaving the body susceptible to invasion. Medications, sickness, chlorine, poor diet, the contraceptive pill, and alcohol are just some of the things that can wipe out your beneficial bacteria. Choosing a probiotic supplement can often be confusing, but make sure it has at least one billion beneficial bacteria and is high in bifidobacteria and lactobacillus. Opt for supplements with enteric-coated capsules, which will keep the bacteria safely inside until it reaches your intestines. Usually one or two capsules daily is enough, but if your beneficial bacteria levels are very low you may need a bigger dose to get them back in balance.

- -

☼ Hot, Healthy, Happy: Take probiotics with antibiotics

If you need to take antibiotics then take probiotics as well, and for a few months afterward. Antibiotic mean 'anti-life', whereas probiotic means 'pro-life.' Many women find they get a thrush outbreak when they take antibiotics, and probiotics should help prevent this happening.

- -

If you have ongoing health problems, then visit www.thefoodpsychologist.com and get a customized supplement program. There you will also find details of the specific brands I recommend, because not all supplements are created equal. When buying supplements remember that cheaper is not always better. Grocery stores and even big chain health food stores favor poor quality, mass-produced supplements. Always be selective and go for high quality supplement companies using pure ingredients. More and more companies are producing supplements without binders, fillers, and synthetic additives.

CAUTION: *Supplements may not be suitable if you are suffering from certain medical conditions, on medications, pregnant, breastfeeding, or planning a pregnancy. Always check with your medical practitioner before introducing supplements.*

On your marks...

Now your kitchen is stocked and loaded, it's time to get started. By the end of this you'll be glowing inside and out, and if you love the new you then keep going. This is your springboard for change. The HHH 21-day diet is designed to free you from discomfort, stress, and unhappiness. Let go of perfection, because it's not achievable, and only ever leads to procrastination and disappointment. The program is not intended to create more stress, but to equip your body, mind, and spirit with the ingredients it needs to achieve the life you want. Becoming obsessive over food is completely the opposite intent and purpose behind this book. If you lose steam halfway through, then just smile and recommit.

Chapter 3

Transition to Hot,
Healthy, Happy

Going cold turkey is not always the easiest way, so give yourself a week of preparation and gently wean yourself off gluten, dairy, stimulants, and processed foods. This will also give you time to dump the junk and restock. Decide when you want to start. If you have an event calendar resembling a socialite's – parties, weddings, and birthdays every other day – then perhaps wait until things quieten down a little. I've lived this way for years; it's simple and doesn't interfere with socializing, but when starting to make changes it is easier if you get your head around the HHH program first and gain confidence before braving the party scene. Get your cupboards loaded with good stuff, your supplements ordered, your juicer and smoothie maker on standby, and your superfoods ready for action. If you need more help, head to www.thefoodpsychologist.com for support in getting started, and we'll have you covered, otherwise this is the plan for the transition week:

♥ Gently take out caffeinated drinks (e.g. coffee, black tea, sodas, and energy drinks). Start by reducing to one cup or glass a day. Check out the coffee alternatives, such as teeccino, barley cup, green teas, and diluted fresh juices, or add a dash of lemon or lime to your glass of water. If you struggle with headaches or find it difficult to get going without a cup of coffee or caffeinated energy drinks, then take 1000mg of tyrosine first thing. (Caution: Tyrosine is not suitable for people with high blood pressure. Always check with your medical practitioner before introducing supplements.) Make your own fizzy juice by mixing fresh fruit juice with carbonated spring water. There are also plenty of alternative energy drinks available, so check out a good quality health food store and have a snoop.

♥ Cut down on the cocktails. Go for organic red wine, and keep it to two glasses a week, max.

♥ Cut down on your meat consumption. If you want to keep fish in your diet, limit it to 2–3 portions a week.

♥ Bring more green into your life. Pull out the juicer and start gyrating those greens. Get adventurous with salads.

♥ Dump processed sugar and refined carbohydrates (e.g. white rice). Now is the time to discover your natural sweetness.

♥ Remove dairy and gluten. Your digestive system will thank you. Switch over to the alternatives and notice your symptoms start to shift.

Imagine your HHH day

On rising

Right Christy, I'm up and ready to rock, what now? Nothing. Give your body breathing space. Then it's time to move. Rebounding is perfect on an empty tummy, so get your bounce on. Yoga or dance would also be awesome. Just 15 minutes of exercise is fine, more if you have the time. Do some dry skin brushing and head for the shower.

Once you're smelling fresh it's time to enjoy a glass of pure filtered water with a squeeze of lemon. If you have trouble with regular bowel movements then start the day with a soaked linseed drink. To make this, add 1dsp of linseeds to a glass of filtered water, soak overnight then drink the entire contents. This could be followed by a cup of herbal tea, green or white tea, or yerba mate.

Breakfast

Ready for something more? It's juice time! Green juices and smoothies are your staples until lunchtime. If you're new to green goodness, don't fret, just check out my formula for green juice and smoothies in the recipes section (see pages 243–246). Experiment, play, taste, savor, and enjoy. Your body, skin, and hair will love you for it. Aim for around 570ml (1 pint) of green juices or smoothies a day, but if you need more then have more. Then try one of these:

- ♥ Big bowl of fresh berries.

- ♥ Free-range egg omelet with fresh chopped kale.

- ♥ A slice or two of sprouted gluten-free bread, topped with delicious nut butter and some sugar-free fruit spread.

- ♥ Alternatively, top a slice of gluten-free bread with lashings of avocado and combine with your choice of hummus, chopped tomato, or a squeeze of agave nectar.

- ♥ A bowl of gluten-free granola topped with dairy-free milk. There are plenty of commercial varieties to choose from, but watch out for added sugar, syrups, glucose, and other unnecessary extras. Even better, make your own (see recipes, page 248).

♥ A bowl of gluten-free porridge oats. Soak organic jumbo oats overnight in some nondairy milk. Heat in the morning and top with fresh berries or grated apple and cinnamon, and a sprinkle of mixed seeds (milled flax, pumpkin, sesame, and sunflower). Fed up with oats? Then check out my millet, quinoa, and buckwheat porridge recipe (see recipes, page 248) for a tasty alternative.

Lunch

Pile your plate with 60–80 percent colorful salad greens and good fats (avocados, cold-pressed oils, nuts, seeds, and other raw deliciousness). Raw veggie pasta, nut pate, cabbage wraps, rice paper wraps, and raw vegetarian sushi are all delicious choices. The remaining 20–40 percent could be healthy and cooked whole foods (slightly sautéed veggies, beans, hummus, tempeh, tofu, gluten-free grains, soup, sweet baked potatoes, or baked butternut squash; add organic butter and high quality sea salt to these). Keep lunch yummy, but not heavy. Here is how to throw something delicious together. Mix and match for endless combinations:

Pick from the following:

♥ **Leafy:** Make a leafy green vegetable salad using kale, spinach, red chard, watercress and/or romaine, or Savoy cabbage, lettuce, rice paper or nori sheets for wraps.

♥ **Grain:** Portion of cooked quinoa, buckwheat, brown rice, or brown rice pasta.

♥ **Starchy:** Small baked sweet potato with butter and sea salt.

Then...

♥ **For crunch:** Add fresh raw chopped red onion, peppers, celery, carrot, tomatoes, grated courgette (zucchini), beansprouts, fennel, asparagus, or lightly sautéed vegetables.

- ♥ **For flavor:** Add fresh herbs such as coriander (cilantro), parsley, basil, rosemary or thyme or try sea salt, wheat-free tamari, apple cider vinegar, Braggs liquid aminos, liquid stevia, nori flakes, dulse flakes, ginger powder, fresh ginger, garlic powder, or fresh garlic.

- ♥ **For good fats:** Dress with cold-pressed seed oils (e.g. hemp seed oil or pumpkin seed oil). Then sprinkle on some seeds (e.g. pumpkin, sunflower, chia, hemp, sunflower, flaxseeds, sesame seeds, or seed butters) or nuts (e.g. almonds, walnuts, macadamias, hazelnuts, pecans, pine nuts or nut butters).

Finish off with:

- ♥ An avocado
- ♥ Bean or lentil burgers
- ♥ Hummus
- ♥ Marinated tofu
- ♥ Tinned chickpeas or mixed beans

If you're still feeling the pressure of social lunches then you could have some fish or eggs with a salad, but ideally this should only make up 20 percent of your meal and the other 80 percent should be green leafy vegetables, non-starchy vegetables, cultured vegetables, and/or ocean vegetables. Don't mix animal products with grains or starchy vegetables (see page 161 for proper food combining).

Mid-afternoon snack

It's 3 p.m. and the vending machine is calling. What do you do? It's snack time! Eating well is not about forgetting snacks. It's about upgrading them! If you prefer grazing on small meals then split your lunch in two and have the second half now. Alternatively, a perfect afternoon pick-me-up is another green juice, green smoothie or berry smoothie with protein powder. Or pick from the following:

- ♥ Brown rice cakes or flax crackers with fresh salsa, guacamole, hummus, or olives

- ♥ Blue corn tortilla chips

- ♥ Popcorn popped in coconut oil

- ♥ Homemade granola bars

- ♥ Gluten-free pancakes

- ♥ A handful of raw nuts or seeds

- ♥ A piece of fresh fruit or some crudités

Check out your local health food store, they're usually packed with raw treats full of live enzymes and nutrients. Yum!

Pre-dinner wind down: Soul food

You're heading home and feeling a little stressed out. How can you make sure the usual old eating patterns don't start? Pre-dinner is usually when most of us hit the snack cupboard. Instead, run yourself a bath and soak. You could add some Epsom salts, apple cider vinegar (see page 166). It's important to ease away the day and relax before you spend time with your family or do something in the evening. Alternatively, you could do a guided meditation. Usually we overeat because our brain is spinning from the day's thoughts, so take some time to chill out before dinner.

Dinner

Now for the best bit. Dinner! Go for the same ratios as at lunch: 60–80 percent colorful salad greens and good fats (avocados, cold-pressed oils, nuts, seeds, and other raw deliciousness). The remaining 20–40 percent should be cooked whole foods. These could include a wide variety of lightly sautéed veggies with gentle protein such as pulses, beans or tofu or fish or served with starchy carbohydrates such as gluten-free grains, quinoa, buckwheat, brown basmati rice, brown rice pasta or sweet baked potatoes/baked butternut squash.

My top tip is to start dinner with a raw salad, which will help digest any cooked foods. It will also mean you're filled with raw alkalizing foods over more acidic foods if you decide to add in some animal protein. For example, if you keep some wild fish in your diet, then stack 60–80 percent of your plate with raw vegetables and 20 percent with fish, with maybe some steamed veggies on the side.

Sipping apple cider vinegar or taking digestive enzymes (HCL and pepsin are not suitable for those suffering from gastritis or ulcers, or those on certain medications) and cultured vegetables may all help with the digestion of animal proteins. Alternatively, have a plant-based dinner. Starchy root vegetables and sweet potatoes are cleaner and easier to digest than grains, but you could include some quinoa, buckwheat, millet, or amaranth with your dinner. Vegetable soups, cabbage wraps, rice paper wraps, and raw sushi are all great options. Please see the recipe section (pages 243–262) for inspiration.

Dessert time

Don't worry, I would never forget dessert! Let me tell you a little secret: I'm a chocoholic, so I like a few squares of dark (70–85 percent cocoa solids) chocolate after dinner. Good quality dark chocolate is also packed with flavonoids, so you can enjoy your treat in the knowledge that it's making you hot, healthy, happy. I also make my own raw chocolates, or how about a scrumptiously sweet sorbet? You can make your own with frozen fruit. For these and lots of other scrumptious recipes, go to the recipe section (see pages 243–264) and find some inspiration.

On your marks, get set, go...

So, for the next 21 days, stuff yourself hot, healthy, happy with plants; eat less meat and more real food; dump the fakes; breathe; do some positive inner parenting; leave the cocktails; don't smoke; turn down stress; build healthy boundaries; burn your to-do list; say 'no' to other people's agendas and 'yes' to your bliss; dump things; slurp your gorgeous green juice; take supplements based on your imbalances; walk in the wild; bathe in the sunshine; take joy seriously; make laughing non-negotiable; and let your inner child play, bend, bounce, cartwheel, skip, dance, paint, make a mess, smile like a three-year-old, and live every day like it's the start of your life and so awesome you can't wait to do it all over again tomorrow. If you're ready to rock and roll, then join me and spend the next 21 days focusing on you.

Chapter 4

21 Days to Hot, Healthy, Happy

Before you start the HHH 21-day diet, here is an important reminder that this is NOT a strict diet program where you have to eat set amounts and portion sizes at specific times. Instead, I've offered suggested menus for the 21 days, and lots of recipes (see pages 243–264). How and whether you use them is up to you. This book is about arming you with information so that you can make empowered choices and create a way of living that works for you.

Every day I will be offering you an affirmation, lifestyle tips, food ideas, and a prayer to get you moving in the right direction. Along the way expect the odd road bump, symptom, or healing crisis, but every day will be different so keep track of your journey in a journal so you can see your progress.

This HHH 21-day diet isn't about missing out, deprivation, or starving. It is about adding flavor, spice, health, and happiness to your everyday menu. You may have a little detox surge at the start, and old cravings may pop up from time to time, but don't worry, hunger is not on the agenda. If you need more help or inspiration then visit me at www.thefoodpsychologist.com for loads more recipes, tests, programs, and tons of free advice.

Day 1

I am strong, confident, bright, and live life on my terms.
I deserve to be healthy and happy.

Hooray! You're here and ready for action. This week is all about becoming balanced in the HHH zone. Stepping your toe out of your comfort zone, while being kind to yourself. Today you'll wave goodbye to coffee, tea, and caffeine, and dump most of the animal products, processed sugar and refined carbohydrates. Start adding in your supplements, superfoods, and protein powders. Slurp your greens and dance in the sunshine, because here we go.

👄 Foodelicious tip

Start every day with a glass of pure filtered water with a squeeze of lemon and/or a linseed soak drink (see page 193). Green juice is another everyday feature of the HHH program. Make a batch of green juice (see recipes, page 243) and separate it into mason jars to keep it fresh and tasty for your afternoon snack.

Fabulous focus

Your thinking over the next 21 days is incredibly vital to your success. Remember, your subconscious doesn't understand negatives, so keep those thoughts peaceful and positive. Call in the language police if necessary. Tell your nagging inner parent to pipe down and practice some positive parenting. Keep your inner talk upbeat, because your body hears every word!

Sassy self-care

It's time to start moving and shaking your body. Dance, bounce, cartwheel, run, walk, whatever floats your boat. How long for? Just

30 minutes, five times a week. Give your lymphatic system an extra boost with dry skin brushing before your morning shower. If you can sweat it out with regular saunas (infrared if possible, see page 87) during this program, even better!

- -

☼ Hot, Healthy, Happy: Green is your new start

Green juices and green smoothies are your one-way ticket to a hot, healthy, happy life. Slurp them every day until noon, and if you need a green recharge in the afternoon then refuel. If you need some more morning oomph then indulge in some of my other sexy suggestions (see recipes, pages 243–248).

- -

Power prayer

Please give me the strength to stay open, curious, and calm. Send me some love in the moments I forget to love myself. Help me live in now and remember that whatever I am doing is just for today; tomorrow will take care of itself.

HOT, HEALTHY, HAPPY... HUNGRY?

Breakfast	Green Goddess Juice (see recipes, page 243) Bowl of berries or an apple
Lunch	Colors of the Rainbow (see recipes, page 251) Hot Smoking Potato (see recipes, page 259)
Snack	A few oatcakes and raw almond butter Instant miso soup
Dinner	Fresh fish and a large dressed salad with stacks of fresh goodies Finish with a few squares of dark chocolate (at least 70–85 percent cocoa solids) or Christy's Secret Raw Chocolate (see recipes, page 264)

Day 2

I love my body enough to give her highly nutritious whole foods and divine thoughts. I trust that she knows how to be naturally healthy and slim.

Well done, superstar, the first day is in the bag! What you dump from your diet is just as crucial as what you include. Every healthy eating plan includes one priceless thing: they all dump the junk food. Clean out your headspace while you're at it, and throw away any nagging trashy talk along with the processed foods.

- -

♡ Foodelicious tip

If you're already missing your daily dose of dairy products, a nondairy milkshake will satisfy those cravings. Throw 1 banana (even try frozen), a glass of nondairy coconut milk, a drizzle of honey, and some chia seeds into the blender and whiz. Wow!

- -

Fabulous focus
Today focus on changing any toxic beliefs you have about nutrition: 'Fat makes you fat,' 'Food is the enemy,' 'I have to starve myself to be thin.' It's time to catch these bad boys in action and kick them where it hurts.

Sassy self-care
Just move. Drop the excuses. Stop putting it off. It only takes 30 minutes, so get it done. How about that little mind workout called meditation? How's that working out for you? Been skipping it? Stop letting your brain talk you out of it. Just turn up and be counted.

Don't worry about getting it perfect, simply breathe and focus on the present moment (if you need a reminder about how to do it, see page 105 in Part III).

- -

☼ Hot, Healthy, Happy: Plan your attack

Failing to plan is planning to fail. Success comes from staying organized. You don't have to stick to the suggested 'meal ideas' but that doesn't mean you shouldn't plan. So dust off those cookbooks, shop, stock, and map it out. Stack the odds for success. Double your meals up so you have less preparation. If you have a fancy juicer you can prepare juices a day or so in advance, too. Think. Plan. Plot. Go.

- -

Power prayer

Let me appreciate my incredible body just as she is now. Give me trust in her. May I know that when I take care of her she looks and feels beautiful.

HOT, HEALTHY, HAPPY... HUNGRY?	
Breakfast	Sunshine Elixir (see recipes, page 245) Gluten-free Porridge (see recipes, page 248) with dairy-free milk
Lunch	Chick Salad (see recipes, page 253)
Snack	Green Goddess Juice (see recipes, page 243) Small handful of raw almonds
Dinner	Posh Quinoa (see recipes, page 259) with a large raw vegetable salad Treat yourself to some Banana Whip (see recipes, page 263)

Day 3

Sometimes when things fall apart
they are actually falling into place.

About to fall off the HHH wagon? Then grab my hand and I'll pull you back up. If you're facing a little health hiccup, stay strong. Pesky symptoms are normal, wise one (so is a full-on healing crisis). Your body is having a spring clean. It'll pass, I promise. Drink your water, slurp your greens, hit the sauna, and keep going, hot stuff. Believe in hot, healthy, happy.

- -

⌣ *Foodelicious tip*

You can buy hummus ready-made (opt for an organic variety if possible), but it's also really easy to make. Drain and rinse a can of chickpeas, then add a little water, a couple of crushed garlic cloves, a couple of tablespoons of tahini paste (to taste), lemon juice, and cumin, then, using a hand-held blender, whiz to a smooth consistency. Add lemon juice, sea salt, and more garlic and cumin if you want. Drizzle with olive oil, a sprinkle of paprika, and a few pine nuts and then dive in.

- -

Fabulous focus

Think about the significant things you've achieved in your life. Focus on how incredible they were when you got to the end, and how great you felt about doing it. Sure, there were little obstacles and setbacks along the way, but you stuck with it and got there. Imagine yourself going through this program; see the 21 days in your head, being ticked off as you successfully make it through another day. Forget perfection, the road to success is paved with persistence. Just keep taking little steps every day.

Sassy self-care

Tonight, give technology the heave-ho. Turn off the tweets, face blank Facebook, and turn off the TV. You'll survive. Pick up that book you've been meaning to read for ages, sit back, and unwind.

- -

☀ Hot, Healthy, Happy: Kick withdrawals

If your favorite coffee cup is calling your name and caffeine withdrawals are kicking in, then try supplementing with tyrosine. This should help pump up your catecholamine levels and curb those caffeine withdrawals. Yippee!

CAUTION: *Tyrosine is not suitable for people with high blood pressure. Always check with your medical practitioner before introducing supplements.*

- -

Power prayer

Allow me to notice how I hold myself back so I can step over the obstacles I place in my path. Give me the courage and strength to walk the road less traveled and not give up on me.

HOT, HEALTHY, HAPPY... HUNGRY?

Breakfast	Rainbow Cocktail (see recipes, page 246) Gluten-free sprouted toast with avocado and hummus
Lunch	Kale and Quinoa Love Affair (see recipes, page 253)
Snack	Ella Berry smoothie (see recipes, page 246)
Dinner	Quinoa Kedgeree (see recipes, page 261) Treat yourself to two Bliss Bombs (see recipes, page 263)

Day 4

*I have the power to be whomever I want.
I create my destiny. I have the confidence
to go after whatever I want in life.*

Now that you're on the road it's time to start thinking about the direction you're heading. Who and what you really want to be. Focus on your emotions and feelings first. Work out how you want to feel then build your goals around those. What steps do you need to take to get you those feelings on a consistent basis?

⌂ Foodelicious tip

Freezing fruit gives you instant desserts. Either whip them up in the blender to make sorbets or simply eat straight from the freezer. Try frozen melon, pineapple, grapes or mixed berries – delicious!

Fabulous focus

Today, think about the kind of life that would make you happy. Forget your culture's ideas about the perfect life. What makes your heart sing? What would make you want to jump out of bed each day? What would life be like if you followed your bliss?

Sassy self-care

Take my visualization master class in Part III (see pages 145–146) and start creating your ultimate dream plan. Throw this into your daily meditation, as you fall off to sleep and whenever you manage to steal a moment to yourself.

☼ *Hot, Healthy, Happy: Get grabby*

Start cutting out snippets from magazines and taking photos that make your heart sing. We will be getting snip happy on Day 18 to create a beautiful vision board, so start collecting now.

Power prayer

Guide me in finding those things that bring me true joy. Allow me to recognize opportunities that come my way, and the courage to grab them with both hands.

HOT, HEALTHY, HAPPY... HUNGRY?

Breakfast	Scrumptious Green Smoothie (see recipes, page 244) Bowl of berries or an apple
Lunch	Brown rice noodles with stir-fried vegetables and tamari Green leafy salad
Snack	Hummus with gluten-free crackers
Dinner	Peace Pots (see recipes, page 258) Instant miso soup Freeze some chopped-up pieces of melon or pineapple for dessert

Day 5

I have the strength to follow anything through. I am a fearless game changer. Stand back world, here I come.

Freaking out because it's nearly the weekend? If Friday night usually signals a binge fest of pizza, fries, and cocktails then don't fear, you can pull this off. Weekends, parties, and nights out are for looking fabulous. Do you look hot when you're stumbling around, garbling nonsense, and throwing up in the bathroom? *Err, no.* Here's my tip. Be a portion princess. Keep your diet clean and nutrient dense and enjoy a little red wine if the moment takes you. Sneak some dark chocolate into your handbag if you're heading out for a meal, or make yourself some popcorn to take to the movies. Forget deprivation, think upgrade. Make this work for you.

- -

⌁ Foodelicious tip

If you are heading out over the weekend and want a flat stomach, stay hydrated with water and herbal teas. Although you may be noticing that cutting gluten out of your diet is already making a difference to your outline.

- -

Fabulous focus

Today, think about people, or even foods, that may need some boundaries. Are you socializing with people that who fun but lead you into unhealthy habits? Be a shining example of someone who follows another path.

Sassy self-care

If you haven't already done so, now is the perfect time to do the building boundaries exercise in Part III (see page 121).

- -

☀ Hot, Healthy, Happy: Don't shout about it

Don't make a fuss about changing your diet or lifestyle. People only really notice when you make a big song and dance about it. It's nobody else's business what you're eating! Be a boundaries babe! Most of the time others are just worried you won't be the same to be around. The truth is, you're going to have more energy, have better mental clarity, be more joyful, and look hot in your skinny jeans. If they aren't interested in a hotter, healthier, happier you, maybe it's time to move on.

- -

Power prayer

Give me the strength and courage to make my own decisions and the confidence to socialize as the real me with my integrity intact. Allow me to inspire others to look after themselves, too.

HOT, HEALTHY, HAPPY... HUNGRY?

Breakfast	Green Guru (see recipes, page 246) Homemade Muesli (see recipes, page 248) with dairy-free milk
Lunch	Rawlicious 'Sushi' (see recipes, page 257)
Snack	Raw veggies (or another hit of Green Guru) Small handful of raw almonds
Dinner	Fresh fish and a large salad with stacks of fresh veggie goodies and a dressing Finish with some Himalayan-salted Popcorn (see recipes, page 263)

Day 6

*I love my tummy and my thighs. I love every bit of me.
My body is happy and healthy. My mind is clear.
Wow, I'm a force to be reckoned with.*

It's time to regroup and reprioritize. If you were caught short of HHH food ideas this week then use your time to restock and refuel. Figure out the best way to make it through next week, Sherlock. You're on a learning curve so be gentle with yourself. Use this time to rethink how you want to eat over the coming week.

- -

☖ Foodelicious tip

If sugar cravings are getting on top of you, try some fermented foods such as apple cider vinegar on your salad, or cultured vegetables with your meals and/or a big swig of Kombucha (an effervescent fermentation of sweetened tea).

- -

Fabulous focus

Make today all about you. Grab your journal and consider any of the challenges that came up for you this week. Stay positive; keep it more inspiring love story than tragic tale. Once you're done head out and do whatever you love to spend time doing. Enjoy the moments of the day and leave rush and worry at home.

Sassy self-care

Get out in nature and run in the wild. Invite your inner child to come out to play. Climb trees, roll in the grass, hunt down caves, and explore. If it's chilly outside, wrap up toasty warm and soak your tootsies in a hot tub when you get home.

- -

☀ Hot, Healthy, Happy: Keep your kitchen HHH

Over the weekend restock for the week ahead. Keep your kitchen brimming with hot, healthy, happy foods. This is the key to success. If you got caught out when you were in the car, or when you were out somewhere last week, then learn from this and get organized so you have foods with you. Wander around the health food store and snag some healthy treats.

- -

Power prayer

Help me to prioritize my health. May I be free and happy. May I be strong and healthy.

HOT, HEALTHY, HAPPY... HUNGRY?	
Breakfast	Sunshine Elixir (see recipes, page 245) Gluten-free sprouted cereal with dairy-free milk
Lunch	An Avocado a Day (see recipes, page 254)
Snack	Celery and carrot sticks with raw cashew nut butter or bean dip or dressing
Dinner	Saucy Portobello Mushrooms (see recipes, page 250) with quinoa Baked Apple Warmer with Cashew Cream (see recipes, page 262)

Day 7

I am free, flowing, carefree, and calm. I find happiness in keeping it simple. I'm a time-management master. I have all the time in the world.

Now you've restocked, your fridge should be brimming with greens. That makes it a perfect day for some extra juicing, so get your whiz on and experiment with some sexy juices or smoothie making. Slurp and savor.

- -

♨ *Foodelicious tip*

Add some cayenne pepper to your morning hot water to get your circulation pumping! Need a boost? Then try some yerba mate; it will definitely put a swing in your step.

- -

Fabulous focus

Are you feeling short of time this week? Are you always running from one place to another? Here's why that isn't going to make life any easier. As I said before being late makes us fat. Why? Because stress makes us fat. There, I said it. Want to be slim and stunning? Be a time-management master. The first step is to prioritize your time; do what matters, and let the rest go.

Sassy self-care

If you've been struggling to meditate then download a guided meditation or chanting audio. This will help you keep on track. Practice for 15–20 minutes every day to give your mind some breathing space.

☀ *Hot, Healthy, Happy: Whiz up a storm in the kitchen*

Freeze bananas, make your own granola, cook soups or stews and freeze them. Make some raw chocolates and granola bars. Get creative and organized for the week ahead. Go online and look around for raw food recipes that make your mouth water. Experiment and expand. If you surround yourself with delicious and healthy options, it makes all the nutrient-challenged processed foods seem unappetizing.

Power prayer

In this crazy world, help me to find calm, to stop overestimating the amount I can do. Help me to give up unnecessary stress and start prioritizing sassy self-care.

HOT, HEALTHY, HAPPY... HUNGRY?

Breakfast	Scrumptious Green Smoothie (see recipes, page 244) Gluten-free granola with dairy-free milk
Lunch	Wholesome Chunky Vegetable Soup (see recipes, page 249) Large raw vegetable salad
Snack	Hummus with gluten-free crackers
Dinner	Mexican Chili (see recipes, page 257) with quinoa Fresh berries with Cashew Cream (see recipes, page 262)

Day 8

*I find beauty is a simpler way of being. Happiness
comes from within, not from the stuff I possess.
I have space and am ready for wonderful things
to come to me. I'm an opportunity magnet.*

Woo hoo, you did it! You made it through the first week. Well done. Maybe it wasn't perfect. Who cares! You're heading in the right direction and that's all that matters. The hardest part is over. You should notice any detox symptoms lessening this week, but if they keep popping up just keep going, because it means you're on your way to being a hot, healthy, happy, skinny-jeans-wearing goddess.

♨ Foodelicious tip

If you're run off your feet today and need to eat in a dash, then a piece of fruit, a small handful of nuts, and a cup of instant miso soup will keep your energy levels high until dinner. Whatever you do, don't skip meals and then binge out later.

Fabulous focus

Yesterday we were thinking about time-management skills. Now it's time to free up some time by having a virtual detox. Are you chained to your e-mail most of the day? Then set an auto-responder and limit yourself to only checking e-mails every three hours or so. Unsubscribe to all the junk mail you never read. Stop multitasking; it's overwhelming, it stresses you out, and, like being late, it makes you fat. Stop snooping on other people on Facebook. Live your life instead of living vicariously through everyone else!

Sassy self-care

Out with the old and in with the new. How about clearing the clutter today? Stop time squeezing by clearing out the time wasting. Once you have detoxed your virtual world move on to clearing your car, rooms, closet, and cupboards. Imagine you could actually find what you need when you need it. Get rid of all the things you never use.

- -

☀ *Hot, Healthy, Happy: Break up with your scales*

If you haven't already, throw out your scales today. This is the perfect time to liberate yourself. Hanging on to clothes you never wear? If you haven't worn it in the last year then give it away.

- -

Power prayer

Help me to make space in my life for the things I really want. Give me the strength to cut the cords with what isn't working.

HOT, HEALTHY, HAPPY... HUNGRY?	
Breakfast	Rainbow Cocktail (see recipes, page 246) Gluten-free sprouted toast with nut butter and sugar-free fruit spread
Lunch	Brown rice pasta with homemade pasta sauce and a green salad
Snack	Bowl of berries
Dinner	Hot Smoking Potato (see recipes, page 259) Colors of the Rainbow (see recipes, page 251) Finish with 3 squares of dark chocolate (at least 70–85 percent cocoa solids) or Christy's Secret Raw Chocolate (see recipes, page 264)

Day 9

I'm letting go. I trust in the universal sorcery to bring me wonderful and happy experiences.

Now that you've been living in the hot, healthy, happy zone for more than a week, you'll hopefully have started to notice that delicious digestive system of yours feeling happier. Is it clearing out or a little clogged up? Stay consistent. If you're still having belly and bowel troubles then recap by reading the chapter on digestion again in Part II (see pages 51–61), and start giving your system some extra oomph; or come over to www.thefoodpsychologist.com and I'll give you a helping hand.

Foodelicious tip

If you're throwing on your sombrero for a fajita night, how about whipping up some fresh guacamole? Throw two peeled and de-stoned avocados, some crushed garlic, and a squeeze of lemon in the blender... whiz... you're done.

Fabulous focus

Notice your stomach today. How do you feel after meals? Are you going to the bathroom regularly? How have your bowel habits been over the last week? Tune in and listen to what your stomach is saying.

Sassy self-care

If you're feeling adventurous then how about spring clearing your colon? You could be carrying around 7lbs (3kg) of extra gunk in there. Give it a clear out and see how much lighter you feel. Book in for a colonic irrigation, or if you're feeling brave, how about a home enema?

☼ Hot, Healthy, Happy: Fire up your food quarantine

If your stomach is bloating after meals try some digestive enzymes or apple cider vinegar, and don't drink water with meals. If you're struggling with constipation then don't forget to include a linseed soak every day.

Power prayer

Sometimes I work myself up over insignificant things. Please help me to see the bigger picture and trust that everything will work out for me.

HOT, HEALTHY, HAPPY... HUNGRY?	
Breakfast	Sunshine Elixir (see recipes, page 245) Gluten-free Porridge (see recipes, page 248) with dairy-free milk
Lunch	Butter Nutty Soup (see recipes, page 250) Skinny Dippers (see recipes, page 254)
Snack	Some oatcakes and hummus
Dinner	Vegetable Fajitas (see recipes, page 256) with a large green salad Finish with a Tropicana Sorbet (see recipes, page 264)

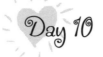

Day 10

*I'm a magnet to incredible delights. I'm chilled.
My body is calm and peaceful.*

How's the stress been? Are you still living in droplet mode or are you acting like a free-flowing wave? The more you can begin to chill out and trust that things are unfolding in the right order, the more you can let go.

- -

⌂ Foodelicious tip

Experiment with milkshakes using dates, frozen bananas, strawberries, cacao powder, and different nondairy milks.

- -

Fabulous focus

Start to notice how often you're in stress response. Now that you've cut all the stimulants and refined sugars from your diet, it's time to get serious about removing any remaining junk-food thoughts. Today, become aware of how your conscious mind is throwing you into stress response. Be a casual observer. Don't engage in it. When you feel your heart start to thud and the anxiety rise, catch the thought, strangle it, and replace it with a positive gem.

Sassy self-care

What about adding some awesome affirmations to your exercise? Get your pump on. Hit a Zumba or dance class and get your sweat on. Moving and shaking is the perfect stress reliever.

☼ *Getting Hot, Healthy, Happy: Eat mindfully*

Take time to notice your food. Eat slowly and be aware of each mouthful. Make sure your brain registers each forkful. When your brain tells you that your stomach is full, then stop eating. This is the secret to not overeating.

Power prayer

Help me to relinquish my iron-tight grip and allow life to unfold naturally. Help me to trust that good things will come to me without force.

HOT, HEALTHY, HAPPY... HUNGRY?	
Breakfast	Green Guru (see recipes, page 246) Homemade Muesli (see recipes, page 248) with dairy-free milk
Lunch	Mineral Rich Nori Omelet (see recipes, page 260) with a large green leafy salad
Snack	Ella Berry Smoothie (see recipes, page 246)
Dinner	Coconut Curry (see recipes, page 255) with brown rice Treat yourself to a Bananarama Milkshake (see recipes, page 247)

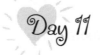

Day 11

*My life starts now. I choose who and what I am today.
I'm ready to release the past and move on to hot,
healthy, happy experiences now.*

Are you finding the same unhelpful stuff rearing its ugly head again and again? Are you living on the disaster rinse-and-repeat cycle? You're building those boundaries, visualizing and praying, and have affirmations coming out of your ears, but the same old thing keeps coming back at you. Don't give up hope, it's just a sign that you need to do things differently and getting your subconscious on board with the hot, healthy, happy game plan is the way forward.

- -

⌚ Foodelicious tip

Stuff your handbag with healthy snacks so you never get caught out. Put some dark chocolate in your bag before you head out for the night, as an after-dinner treat.

- -

Fabulous focus

Today, focus on any negative patterns of behavior and ask yourself why you keep facing the same problems over and over again. What are you getting from these? Why are you attracting these to you?

Sassy self-care

Check out the exercise for schmoozing a stubborn subconscious in Part III (see pages 143–144) and dissolving the disaster rinse-and-repeat cycle. Get cozy with your subconscious and help her bring new, exciting experiences into your life and break the old patterns that are holding you back.

- -

☼ Hot, Healthy, Happy: Become a smoothie queen

Get creative with your smoothies today. Throw in some superfoods and have fun. Let your inner child experiment, and create some love potions.

- -

Power prayer

Allow me to see what is holding me back. Give me the strength to let go of my past and the realization that my biography is not my destiny.

HOT, HEALTHY, HAPPY... HUNGRY?

Breakfast	Green Goddess Juice (see recipes, page 243) Gluten-free toast with cashew nut butter
Lunch	Open-Face Avocado Sandwich (see recipes, page 255) Instant miso soup
Snack	Crudités and bean dip or hummus
Dinner	Fresh fish with a large leafy green salad and dressing Freeze some pineapple and melon chunks for dessert

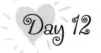

Day 12

*I have the incredible ability to move past
my fears. I choose how I feel and respond.
My live is abundant and full of joy.*

Yesterday we were thinking about negative patterns and ongoing issues that keep reappearing time and time again. If they stem from your childhood you may be filtering beliefs through a wounded and afraid inner child. Have you reconnected with her recently?

- -

♨ Foodelicious tip

Homemade soups (e.g. broccoli, carrot, or vegetable) are really easy to make. Start by sautéing a chopped onion, some crushed garlic, and a couple of small white potatoes (cubed and par-boiled) in a little olive oil. Next add your chosen vegetables plus a few spices or herbs, and pour over enough vegetable stock (use a gluten-free stock cube) to just cover the vegetables. Simmer until the vegetables are lightly cooked and then pass through a blender and season to taste. Easy!

- -

Fabulous focus

Think about how much you've grown over the years: all the things that have worked out wonderfully, and all those times when you felt afraid but triumphed. Give yourself a pat on the back for all the good things you have accomplished that you've never really taken the time to give yourself credit for.

Sassy self-care

If you have some time today, use it to reconnect with your inner child. Follow the exercise for reconnecting with your inner child in Part III (see pages 135–136). Have your inner parent create some beautiful positive messages to give to your inner child. Then take her out to play.

- -

☼ Hot, Healthy, Happy: Get your beauty sleep.

How is that beauty sleep coming along? Try hitting the hay by 10:30 p.m., reading and eyes shut by 11 p.m. Turn your bedroom into a sleeping haven. Invest in blackout blinds, upgrade your bedding, and clear out all electromagnetic disturbances from TVs, radios, phones, etc. Let your mind freewheel through dreamland in peace.

- -

Power prayer

Help me to release the pain from my past and heal my scared inner child. Let me give her the love and strength she needs to grow up to be a happy adult.

HOT, HEALTHY, HAPPY... HUNGRY?	
Breakfast	Scrumptious Green Smoothie (see recipes, page 244)
Lunch	Wholesome Chunky Vegetable Soup (see recipes, page 249) Kale and Quinoa Love Affair (see recipes, page 253)
Snack	Apple or pear Small handful of almonds
Dinner	Brown rice pasta and fresh homemade pasta sauce with a large leafy green salad Finish with some yummy Banana Whip (see recipes, page 263)

Day 13

*I have the capability to deal with anything
that comes my way. Every day, I am growing.*

Did your inner child work bring up some unexpected feelings? Then it's time to let them all out. Release them any way you choose: scream and shout – whatever it takes to vent them. Punch some pillows. Hit a kickboxing class and feel the fury. If you're sad then pop on a weepy movie; let the tears fall, pour your heart into a journal, or share with a trusted friend. Allow yourself time to feel.

- -

♨ Foodelicious tip

Try adding some chia seeds to your green smoothies; they are great for aiding your digestive system.

- -

Fabulous focus

Notice your emotions today and what comes up for you. Think about why you feel a certain way. If a negative emotion lifts its head, honor it and be curious: 'Oh hello, why are you here?'

Sassy self-care

Let out all those emotions by dancing naked. Finish with a long hot soak in the tub to relax those muscles.

- -

☀ Hot, Healthy, Happy: Emotional eating

Is emotional eating swallowing you whole? Drop the guilt... it happens to us all. But you have a choice. Instead of cookies and chips, splurge on HHH foods. An even better option would be to deal with the problem by bringing your mind into the present: meditate for ten minutes, calm your body and focus your breath, take a walk in nature, put on your running shoes and pound it out of your system. Whatever helps you to release and let go, just do it... work up an appetite for dinner.

- -

Power prayer

Give me the courage to tune in to what I feel and honor what comes up for me in life. To respect where I am on my journey.

HOT, HEALTHY, HAPPY... HUNGRY?	
Breakfast	Rainbow Cocktail (see recipes, page 246) Sprouted gluten-free cereal with dairy-free milk
Lunch	Broccoli soup Large green leafy salad
Snack	Bowl of berries
Dinner	Coconut Curry (see recipes, page 255) with quinoa Finish with a few squares of dark chocolate (70–80 percent cocoa solids) or Christy's Secret Raw Chocolate (see recipes, page 264)

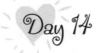

Day 14

By choosing to forgive I am freeing myself from emotional and physical blocks. I have let go of my past and am excited about my future. For today I can forgive.

Brace yourself because I am going to pull out the 'F' word. Forgiveness. When we start to let go of feelings this can seem like an impossible hurdle. Are you holding on to grudges? Want to free yourself? Pick peace. This is the road to health and happiness. You don't need to buddy up with your bullies, sleep with the enemy, or even dismiss any abuse. Instead, you just need to put you first. Negative emotions block your flow. Releasing them is vital for wellness. Maybe it's your body you need to forgive. Reframe and refresh. Learn what it's trying to teach you. Allow yourself to forgive your friends and family – and your thighs and tummy. Forgive you.

- -

⏻ Foodelicious tip

Want a great evening snack or something refreshing on a hot day, then try making some homemade ice lollies (popsicles). Add freshly squeezed juices to a plastic lolly (popsicle) maker (you can get PBA-free versions) then pop them in the freezer. Alternatively, freeze a juice smoothie in an ice-cube tray and then blend the cubes. Voila, instant sorbet! Top flavors to try include cherry, mango, and orange.

- -

Fabulous focus

Compile a list of all the people and situations, and every part of you that you need to forgive.

Sassy self-care

Schedule yourself some play time. Get bouncing on the trampoline. Dance to your favorite tunes. Take a bike ride. Just 30 minutes. Done and dusted.

☼ Hot, Healthy, Happy: Have a fire session

Write down the wrongs that have happened to you in your life on a little piece of paper. Acknowledge each one then release each one by setting it on fire. Watch it go up in smoke. *Poof!*

Power Prayer

Give me the strength to move past my past and to forgive and release the pain.

HOT, HEALTHY, HAPPY... HUNGRY?	
Breakfast	Green Goddess Juice (see recipes, page 243) Sprouted gluten-free toast with avocado or cashew nut butter
Lunch	Peace Pots (see recipes, page 258)
Snack	Hummus and gluten-free crackers
Dinner	Fresh fish with lightly steamed vegetables Banana Whip (see recipes, page 263)

Day 15

I am madly in love with how incredible I feel.
I'm so happy with my life today.

You know that what you eat can affect your biochemistry and have you spurting out happy messengers. You're more than halfway through now and stocked to the brim with good-mood foods. Suck up these good feelings and start to embrace the things you love in your life.

☚ *Foodelicious tip*

Cook a batch of soup, portion it out, freeze it and hey presto, you have some quick lunches for mid-week.

Fabulous focus

Focus today on all the joy and goodness that's in your life. What brings you happiness and joy? Lighten your load by loving your life more.

Sassy self-care

Write yourself a list of everything you love and what makes you feel gratitude. Love will make you glow. Invite love round for a green juice. Begin to look for the beauty and blessings. They're all around you.

- -

☀ Hot, Healthy, Happy: Shop girl!

Get your kitchen locked and loaded for another awesome week. Keep your love brimming as you hit the grocery store. Look for new, amazing, functional foods you have yet to fall in love with. Bring them home, share the love with family and friends and then devour.

- -

Power prayer

Give me the miracle mindset and allow me to notice all the incredible things in my life.

HOT, HEALTHY, HAPPY... HUNGRY?	
Breakfast	Green Goddess Juice (see recipes, page 243) Bowl of mixed berries
Lunch	Hearty Bean Soup (see recipes, page 249) 'Peanut' Satay Salad (see recipes, page 252)
Snack	Green Goddess Juice (see recipes, page 243) Small handful of almonds
Dinner	Saucy Portobello Mushrooms (see recipes, page 250) with a large leafy green salad and quinoa Finish with two Bliss Bombs (see recipes, page 263)

Day 16

*I am perfect at persisting. As long as
I keep going, I will get there.*

The road to success is always hilly. It isn't a straight shot upward. When moments falter and time stands still, don't panic because this is the time to breathe and embrace the peace. Allow yourself time to regroup before the next spurt.

- -

⌣ *Foodelicious tip*

Sprinkle mixed seeds on your salads for extra oomph. You could even toast them a little first for extra deliciousness.

- -

Fabulous focus

Notice your energy today. Do you have a natural flow? If you think it needs a boost then focus on getting plenty of nutrients, oxygen, and sunshine. These will give you a natural lift.

Sassy self-care

Pump some iron and reward yourself by sinking into an Epsom salts or apple cider vinegar bath after your workout.

- -

☼ *Hot, Healthy, Happy: Are you fermentation fabulous?*

Have you tried any fermented foods or seaweeds yet? Where's that sense of adventure? Be brave and get cracking, there's no better time than the present. Fermented foods such as apple cider vinegar, seaweeds and tamari, Kombucha, and even pre-prepared cultured vegetables, are widely available and really add some zing to your meals and your digestion.

- -

Power Prayer

Help me to stay consistent. Even when I feel like I'm stuck, give me trust that things are happening just as they should be.

HOT, HEALTHY, HAPPY... HUNGRY?

Breakfast	Sunshine Elixir (see recipes, page 245) Gluten-free Porridge (see recipes, page 248) with dairy-free milk
Lunch	Mineral Rich Nori Omelet (see recipes, page 260) and a large green leafy salad
Snack	A few oatcakes and almond butter
Dinner	Vegetable Fajitas (see recipes, page 256) and a leafy green salad Finish with a few squares of dark chocolate (at least 70–85 percent cocoa solids) or Christy's Secret Raw Chocolate (see recipes, page 264)

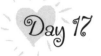

Day 17

*I'm incredible at communicating my knowledge
and experience clearly to others.*

You've been on this journey for a couple of weeks now. Ready
to share the love? Then start spreading the word. Share the hot,
healthy, happy recipe. Share your juicing jewels. Make some raw
chocolates (see recipe, page 262) and offer them around. Have
some friends over for dinner.

- -

○ Foodelicious tip

Ever tried sprouts? Pick some up at your local grocery store and toss
them on top of a salad. Sprouts are packed full of cancer-fighting
flavonoids and super good for you. If you're feeling adventurous then
grow your own. All you need are some beans, pulses, or seeds; jam jars;
plastic wrap; and water. For more information, pop on over to www.
thefoodpsychologist.com and I will guide you through the steps.

- -

Fabulous focus

Forge the path and make it easier for others to follow.

Sassy self-care

Give your skin a beautiful extended dry brush, enjoy a hot shower
then smear up with coconut oil. Bliss.

- -

☀ Hot, Healthy, Happy: Inspiring others

When giving others a taste of new dishes, keep it simple. Remember that most people are used to ramped-up sweet, salty, and fatty foods. So choose options that use natural healthy fats, natural sugars, or sea salt. Play to their taste buds while keeping the ingredients healthy and delicious. Give them something they can ease in with and then watch them flourish.

- -

Power prayer

Enable me to share my experience in a way that others understand. Let me be passionate without overwhelming them. Help me to share with patience and understanding

HOT, HEALTHY, HAPPY... HUNGRY?	
Breakfast	Scrumptious Green Smoothie (see recipes, page 244)
Lunch	Hearty Bean Soup (see recipes, page 249) Rawlicious 'Sushi' (see recipes, page 257)
Snack	Bowl of berries
Dinner	Fresh fish with a large green leafy salad Baked Apple Warmer and Cashew Cream (see recipes, page 262)

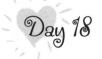

Day 18

I am glowing from the inside out.

Do you have enough light in your life? Good mood foods will have you brimming with serotonin. What about the shiny happy people, are you surrounding yourself with them? I hope you've been slurping those greens and flooding your system with a morning glass of sunshine.

♨ Foodelicious tip

Investigate the chilled cabinets at your local grocery store to find some ready-made stars that you can just take home, heat, and enjoy. There are some great new organic food companies out there making fantastic veggie soups, stews, and sauces without any junk, dairy, or gluten. Great for busy days or when you don't feel like cooking.

Fabulous focus

Become conscious of how much time you spend inside. Schedule yourself sunshine and fresh-air breaks throughout the day. Breathe in the natural environment and let it fill every nook and cranny.

Sassy self-care

Time to create your vision board. Start pinning up all those gorgeous images and snippets you have been collecting.

☼ *Hot, Healthy, Happy: Shine some light into your life.*

Try to spend at least ten minutes every day in the sunshine. If you live where there's little light then invest in a light box and sit it next to you as you read or work at your computer.

Power prayer

Remind me that my body needs light, love, and oxygen to keep it glowing.

HOT, HEALTHY, HAPPY... HUNGRY?	
Breakfast	Scrumptious Green Smoothie (see recipes, page 244)
Lunch	Mexican Chili (see recipes, page 257) with a green salad
Snack	Crudités and hummus
Dinner	Hot Smoking Potato (see recipes, page 259) An Avocado a Day (see recipes, page 254) Bowl of fresh berries

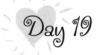

Day 19

I'm surrounded by people who can support me.
I am loved. I am safe. I can figure anything out.

One of the most powerful lessons I learned during my journey was to keep learning. How my body worked. How my mind worked. How to prepare food. How to look after myself. Even now, I am constantly expanding and growing. This is how we find fulfillment – we grow and we give back to others. If your body still has some kinks to smooth out then keep going. Stay curious. Read. Investigate. Explore.

- -

♻ Foodelicious tip

Don't forget to add some chopped fresh herbs to your soups, salads, juices, and smoothies; they are packed with nutrients and give great flavor.

- -

Fabulous focus

Think about the resources you have at your disposal for making life easier. Are there others around you who can help you with ongoing issues? Do you need more support?

Sassy self-care

Pamper yourself. What would you love to do? Have a massage? Reiki session? Spend an hour in a flotation tank? Then do it.

- -

☀ Hot, Healthy, Happy: Take the guesswork out of your health

If your body is confusing you with ongoing symptoms then have a look at testing with the functional medicine labs. I found these tests were the missing piece of the puzzle for my recovery. Take the guesswork out of it. Visit www.thefoodpsychologist.com for more information.

- -

Power prayer

Help me to keep growing and learning about me. Give me the courage to be honest with myself and ask for help when I need it.

HOT, HEALTHY, HAPPY... HUNGRY?

Breakfast	Rainbow Cocktail (see recipes, page 246) Gluten-free toast with cashew nut butter and sugar-free fruit spread
Lunch	Marinated/smoked tofu and a leafy green salad
Snack	A few oatcakes with almond butter.
Dinner	Tomato and Balsamic Baked Cod (see recipes, page 260) and a green salad Bananarama Milkshake (see recipes, page 247)

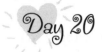

Day 20

*I am a magnet to delicious and beautiful relationships.
We love and care for each other. We respect one
another and help keep each other on track.*

You're almost there. How incredible are you! How are you feeling? Exhilarated? Inspired? Full of green beans (*literally*)? As you near the end of your journey reflect on your progress and how far you've come. Appreciate the changes you've made and the distance you've traveled.

- -

⌂ *Foodelicious tip*

Ever tried maca powder? You can pick it up from your local health food store and it tastes yummy. If your adrenals are under the weather due to stress or lack of sleep, throw this into your smoothies and raw chocolates to give them an extra health boost.

- -

Fabulous focus

Create a power posse of hot, healthy, happy heroines. Cheer each other on. Find strength in numbers. It's much easier to keep this crazy show on the road when you're riding it with other fierce and fabulous women.

Sassy self-care

Is it time for a makeover? Are you stocked up on new natural make-up? What about trying a new look? Some red lipstick and a sparkle in your eye? What about a new hairdo? Hit the hairdressers and have her shimmy up something fabulous.

☼ Hot, Healthy, Happy: Get your glow on

There are some incredible self-tanning creams that don't contain any junk. Give yourself a gorgeous gunk-free glow to show off your super-slimmed thighs!

Power prayer

Allow me to attract those who can help me continue on this incredible journey.

HOT, HEALTHY, HAPPY... HUNGRY?	
Breakfast	Scrumptious Green Smoothie (see recipes, page 244)
Lunch	Rawlicious 'Sushi' (see recipes, page 257)
Snack	Apple or pear
Dinner	Brown rice pasta with a homemade pasta sauce and a green salad Himalayan-salted Popcorn (see recipes, page 263)

Day 21

Today I'm a miracle maker.
I can do anything I set my mind to.

Whoa! You did it. I'm giving you a full on, clapping, cheering, standing ovation. Well done, starshine, you're a force to be reckoned with. As you move forward remember this isn't about absolutes. You just need to cruise in the hot, healthy, happy zone most of the time. Keep yourself brimming with plant-fuelled, alkalizing goodness. Leave the stress and mess alone.

- -

🖐 Foodelicious tip

Don't be afraid of fat, salt, or sweetness. Instead, upgrade to Himalayan or Celtic sea salt, raw plant fats, and natural sweeteners; they're incredible.

- -

Fabulous focus

Live in and enjoy the now. Take each day, hour, and minute as it comes. Forget worrying about the past, you can't change it – life is happening now, so enjoy every moment of it. You can handle the future when it comes.

Sassy self-care

Whatever you want you deserve it, superstar!

☼ Hot, Healthy, Happy: You're here!

You've changed your food, your mood, and your mind. Shaken that booty, meditated, laughed, loved, prayed, rocked it with your inner child, affirmed and crafted up some incredible visualizations for your sassy subconscious. But what if you still don't believe in your wonderful self? Then just keep hanging on in there. You've got to see it first. To be a hot, healthy, happy woman you have to act like one. So keep going through the motions. Show your subconscious how it's done and she'll catch on; she's super smart. Back chat those negative thoughts and stamp them out with visualizations and promises of peace. Keep your positive parenting up. I believe in you. I love you. I think you're incredible. Thank you from the bottom of my heart for taking this wild ride with me and I'm thrilled you did.

Power prayer

Remind me when I forget that I'm amazing just as I am. Let me stay true to me and face my future with joy, creativity, integrity, and passion.

HOT, HEALTHY, HAPPY... HUNGRY?	
Breakfast	Sunshine Elixir (see recipes, page 245) Gluten-free granola with dairy-free milk
Lunch	Marinated/smoked tofu salad Instant miso soup
Snack	Green Goddess Juice (see recipes, page 243) Small handful of almonds
Dinner	Wild fish and a large green leafy salad. Treat yourself with a Tropicana Sorbet (see recipes, page 264)

Chapter 5
Hot, Healthy, Happy Recipes

Need some inspiration? Get excited, experiment, and enjoy. The fabulous thing about natural foods is they're all unique. Don't get too pernickety about the measurements and amounts. Be bold, brave, and use your flair. Add an extra handful of veggies or a pinch of spices; adjust, and play. Make them appeal to your taste buds. Play with the flavor and consistency. Make them your own.

Juices, smoothies, and drinks

Green Goddess Juice

Juicy base
Start with a cucumber – they're super juicy (if you can't afford to go organic then simply remove the skin, then juice). You could also add some celery sticks.

Green leafy goodness
Now you want to add some green leafy vegetables. Pick one of the following:

Romaine lettuce head

Handful of kale

Handful of spinach

Handful of red chard

Flavor

Add 1 whole lemon (including the rind) and 2.5cm (1in) of peeled ginger root to give your taste buds a kick.

Sweetness

Add 1–2 green apples or, if you want to avoid fruit, you could use stevia.

Extra oomph

A handful of herbs, such as coriander (cilantro) or parsley, are awesome, as are superfood powders (e.g. spirulina, chlorella, barley grass, wheatgrass, etc.) although go easy on these because they affect the taste.

Push all the ingredients through a juicer and separate into airtight containers. Drink throughout the morning.

❤ ❤ ❤

Scrumptious Green Smoothie

Green smoothies are just as easy as green juices to make. Ingredients are similar, but you need a high-powered blender instead.

Juicy base and green leafy goodness

Follow the first two steps for making Green Goddess Juice and then add the following:

Sweetness

In the beginning, green smoothies usually taste best with sweeter tropical fruits, so you might want to add:

1 medium mango (peel and remove the stone)

1 banana (fresh or frozen)

½ pineapple (fresh or frozen)

Or try fruits with less sugar such as:

1–2 handfuls of berries (strawberries, blueberries, raspberries, etc.)

1–2 green apples

1–2 pears

In the beginning you might need more sweetness, so you could start with 60 percent fruit to 40 percent greens. As you get used to smoothies, go for 60–80 percent greens and 20–40 percent fruit.

Extra oomph
Try one or two of the following:

A handful of fresh herbs (e.g. coriander/cilantro or parsley)

A sprinkle of superfood powder (e.g. spirulina, chlorella, barley grass, wheatgrass, maca, lucuma, or cacao)

An avocado to make it creamy and delicious

Some gelatinous seeds (e.g. chia or flaxseed)

A drizzle of cold-pressed oil (e.g. flaxseed, hemp, pumpkin seed oil)

Sunshine Elixir
Serves 1

1 romaine lettuce head

1 handful kale

1 cucumber

1 whole lemon

2.5cm (1in) fresh ginger, peeled (or to taste)

1–2 green apples.

Juice the vegetables and the fruits one at a time. Pour into a glass and slurp away!

❤ ❤ ❤

Rainbow Cocktail
Serves 1

1 handful kale

1 whole medium beetroot, peeled

1 romaine lettuce head

1 cucumber

1 whole lemon

2.5cm (1in) fresh root ginger, peeled (to taste)

1–2 green apples

Juice the vegetables and fruits one at a time. Pour the juice into a glass and enjoy the energy boost!

♥♥♥

Green Guru
Serves 1

1 cucumber

1 avocado

1 mango

2 handfuls spinach

120–240ml (4–8fl oz) water or freshly pressed apple juice

Whiz all the ingredients in a high-powered blender until smooth and serve immediately.

♥♥♥

Ella Berry Smoothie
Serves 1

1 scoop hemp protein powder

2 handfuls mixed fresh berries

Drizzle of apple juice or water to thin

Throw all the ingredients in a high-powered blender and whiz until smooth, then enjoy.

❤❤❤

Bananarama Milkshake
Serves 1

1 banana

2 medjool dates, de-stoned

120–240ml (4–8fl oz) coconut milk

1dsp hazelnut butter

Sprig of fresh mint (for decoration)

Whiz all the ingredients in a high-speed blender until smooth and serve over ice with a sprig of mint.

❤❤❤

Almond Milk
Makes approximately 1.2L (2 pints)

200g (8oz) organic raw almonds

1tsp sea salt

720ml (1¼ pints) filtered water

1tsp alcohol-free pure vanilla extract

4tbsps agave nectar or maple syrup or 4–6 dates, pitted and finely chopped

Place the almonds in a bowl, cover with water and the sea salt, and leave for about 12 hours. Rinse the nuts several times and put them and the freshly filtered water in a high-speed blender and whiz until they have a smooth consistency. Strain the milk with a nut bag or sieve with small holes. Sweeten with the vanilla extract and agave nectar. Store in a glass jar in the refrigerator (consume within 2 days).

Breakfast cereals

Homemade Muesli
Makes 5 servings

150g (5oz) gluten-free rolled oats

75g (3oz) dried cranberries

15g (½oz) raw coconut chips

20g (¾oz) raisins

50g (2oz) pumpkin/sesame/sunflower seeds

150g (5oz) macadamia nuts

200ml (6fl oz) almond, coconut, or oat milk to cover

1tsp vanilla extract

Place the oats, cranberries, coconut chips, raisins, and seeds in a bowl. Blend the macadamia nuts with the nut milk and vanilla extract then pour over the dry ingredients. Cover and refrigerate overnight. Serve with grated apple or fresh fruit of your choice, a drizzle of honey, and a splash more milk to moisten if required.

❤❤❤

Gluten-free Porridge
Serve 2

2tbsps millet flakes

1tbsp quinoa flakes

1tbsp buckwheat flakes

240ml (8fl oz) nut milk

1dsp maple syrup, agave nectar or honey

Soak the flakes in 120ml (4fl oz) of nut milk overnight. Then heat the millet, quinoa, and buckwheat flakes, adding the remaining nut milk for 5 minutes on a low heat until the flakes are soft. Divide into two bowls, drizzle sweetness on top and serve immediately.

❤❤❤

Superfood soups and salads

Wholesome Chunky Vegetable Soup
Serves 2

1 broccoli head, chopped

1 courgette (zucchini), chopped

1 leek, chopped

8 mushrooms, chopped

5 celery stalks, chopped

1 red onion, chopped

6 carrots, chopped

400g (14oz) can of brown lentils, drained and rinsed

1.5L (2½pints) vegetable stock (yeast-free stock cube)

Pinch of curry powder (to taste)

Pinch of mixed herbs and sea salt (to taste)

1tbsp fresh coriander (cilantro), chopped

Add all the ingredients except the coriander to a large pot and bring to the boil, simmer until the carrots are semi-soft. Serve with a sprinkle of fresh coriander.

❤ ❤ ❤

Hearty Bean Soup
Serves 2

2tsps olive oil

1 onion, roughly chopped

5 garlic cloves, peeled and chopped

2 celery stalks, chopped

½ leek, finely chopped

½ red pepper, chopped

½ yellow pepper, chopped

1dsp dried oregano

1tbsp fresh basil, chopped

400g (14oz) can of chopped tomatoes

1tbsp fresh parsley, chopped

240ml (8fl oz) vegetable stock (yeast-free stock cube)

400g (14oz) can of mixed beans or kidney beans, drained and rinsed

Heat the olive oil in a large pan and sauté the onion and garlic for 2–3 minutes. Then add the celery, leek, and peppers and cook for another 4–5 minutes. Add the oregano and tomatoes and cook for a further 5 minutes. Add the vegetable stock, parsley, and basil and cook for a further 5 minutes, then add the beans. Sprinkle with a little more chopped parsley, serve, and enjoy.

❤❤❤

Butter Nutty Soup

1 tbsp olive oil

1 butternut squash, peeled and chopped

1 large onion, peeled and chopped

1–2 tsp paprika

750ml (1½ pints) vegetable stock

Heat 1 tbsp of oil in a large pan. Add the squash and onion, and sauté for a few minutes. Stir in paprika and cook gently for 5 minutes. Add enough vegetable stock to cover the vegetables and simmer until soft. Allow to cool, then liquidize. Add extra stock to thin to desired consistency.

❤❤❤

Saucy Portobello Mushrooms
Serves 2

1–2tbsps olive oil

4 Portobello mushrooms, roughly chopped

1dsp honey/agave nectar/maple syrup

1tbsp tamari

1 head celery, finely chopped

½ cucumber, chopped

1 tomato, chopped

2 spring onions (scallions), chopped

1tbsp basil, chopped

½ lemon, juiced

Pinch of mixed herbs and sea salt to season (to taste)

Heat the olive oil gently in a pan. Add the mushrooms and sauté with the honey and tamari for 3–4 minutes. Mix the remaining ingredients in a bowl, then season and top with the mushrooms. Serve with quinoa or a mixed herbs and sea salt, leafy green salad.

♥ ♥ ♥

Colors of The Rainbow
Serves 2

2 avocados, chopped

4 sundried tomatoes, chopped

½ medium red cabbage, finely chopped

100g (4oz) fennel, finely chopped

1 carrot, finely chopped

½ red pepper, finely chopped

½ yellow pepper, finely chopped

1 red onion, finely chopped

1 celery stick, finely chopped

1 garlic clove, peeled and crushed

2tbsps balsamic dressing

1tbsp fresh coriander (cilantro)

Drizzle of agave/honey or a few drops of stevia

Pinch of mixed herbs and sea salt to season (to taste)

Squeeze of fresh lemon juice

Mix all the ingredients together and serve.

♥ ♥ ♥

'Peanut' Satay Salad
Serves 2

For the salad:

400g (14oz) can of chickpeas

2 handfuls beansprouts

2 carrots, peeled and finely sliced

½ yellow pepper, finely sliced

2 spring onions (scallions), thinly sliced

1 small red onion, thinly sliced

120ml (4fl oz) 'Peanut' Satay Sauce (see below)

For the sauce:

1tbsp cashew nut butter

1tbsp olive oil

1tbsp fresh coriander (cilantro)

1tbsp honey (if possible, opt for raw honey)

1 garlic clove, chopped

2.5cm (1in) ginger, peeled and minced

Blend all the ingredients for the sauce together in a high-powered blender. Mix all the salad ingredients together and dress with 'Peanut' Satay Sauce. Delicious!

♥ ♥ ♥

Chick Salad
Serve 2

For the salad:
400g (14oz) can organic chickpeas, drained and rinsed
1 red pepper, finely chopped
1 yellow pepper, finely chopped
1 small red onion, finely chopped
3 spring onions (scallions), chopped
2 tbsp of fresh coriander (cilantro), chopped
40g (1½ oz) fresh rocket

For the dressing:
1 tbsp hemp oil
1 tbsp fresh orange juice
1 dsp wholegrain mustard
Combine ingredients in bowl and drizzle over the dressing.

♥ ♥ ♥

Kale and Quinoa Love Affair
Serves 2

100g (4oz) uncooked quinoa
240ml (8fl oz) vegetable stock (yeast-free stock cube)
2 large tomatoes, finely chopped
2 avocados, chopped
4 handfuls kale, finely chopped
110g (4oz) parsley, finely chopped
1tbsp balsamic vinegar
1 lemon, juiced
Few drops of stevia (to taste)
Pinch of mixed herbs and sea salt to season (to taste)

Cook the quinoa in the vegetable stock according to the packet instructions. Add the cooked quinoa to a bowl and then add the remaining ingredients. Mix together gently, season, and enjoy.

♥ ♥ ♥

An Avocado a Day
Serves 2

4 handfuls kale, chopped

4 sun-dried tomatoes, finely chopped

2 avocados

1tbsp of fresh coriander (cilantro), chopped

1tbsp hemp oil

1tbsp balsamic vinegar

Pinch of mixed herbs and sea salt to season (to taste)

Mix all the ingredients together in a bowl, and season with the mixed herbs and sea salt. Serve immediately and enjoy.

♥ ♥ ♥

Skinny Dippers
Makes 2

1–2tbsp cashew nut butter

2 large Savoy cabbage leaves

1 red pepper, finely sliced

1 small red onion, finely sliced

1 carrot, finely sliced

1tbsp of fresh sprouts (e.g. sprouted chickpeas, mung beans, aduki beans, sunflower seeds, etc.)

1tbsp fresh coriander (cilantro)

1tbsp tamari

Smear the nut butter onto each of the cabbage leaves. Place the pepper, onion, carrot, sprouts and coriander in the center of the cabbage leaves and dress with tamari. Wrap the cabbage leaves around the vegetables and devour.

❤❤❤

Open-Face Avocado Sandwich

Serves 2

2 slices of gluten-free, buckwheat bread, toasted

1 tbsp of Dijon mustard

1 avocado, sliced

1 tomato

2 tbsp of radish and alfalfa sprouts

1 tbsp of fresh coriander (cilantro), chopped

Sea salt to season

Toast the bread to soften it, and spread with the Dijon mustard. Add the avocado and tomato, and top with the sprouts and coriander. Season to taste with sea salt.

❤❤❤

Hearty main courses

Coconut Curry

Serves 2

2tsps coconut oil

1 onion, finely chopped

2.5cm (1in) fresh root ginger, peeled and chopped

1 garlic clove, peeled and crushed

1 butternut squash, peeled and chopped

400g (14oz) can of coconut milk

½ yeast-free vegetable stock cube, crumbled

2tsps garam masala

1tsp ground coriander (cilantro)

2tsps ground cumin

1tsp ground turmeric

8 shitake mushrooms, finely chopped

1tbsp fresh coriander (cilantro), finely chopped

1tbsp fresh parsley, finely chopped

Heat the coconut oil in a pan and gently sauté the onion, ginger, and garlic for a couple of minutes. Add the butternut squash and sauté for a further 5 minutes. Add the coconut milk, stock cube, garam masala, ground coriander, cumin, and turmeric and cook for another 5 minutes. Add the shitake mushrooms and fresh herbs and simmer until the butternut squash is tender. Serve with quinoa.

❤❤❤

Vegetable Fajitas
Serves 2

1tbsp olive oil

1 garlic clove, minced

1 red onion, chopped

2.5cm (1in) fresh root ginger, peeled and minced

1 broccoli head, chopped

1 carrot, chopped

8 shitake mushrooms, chopped

1 red pepper, deseeded and chopped

240ml (8fl oz) vegetable stock (yeast-free stock cube)

2tbsps tamari

2 nori sheets

Mixed herbs and sea salt to season (to taste)

Heat the olive oil and gently sauté the onion, garlic, and ginger for 2–3 minutes. Add the broccoli, carrot, red pepper, shitake mushrooms, vegetable stock, and tamari, and steam fry (covered) over a low heat until the vegetables are slightly softened. Divide the mixture between the nori sheets, season to taste, and serve.

♥ ♥ ♥

Rawlicious 'Sushi'
Makes 2

2 parsnips, chopped

1tbsp tahini

2 nori sheets

1 carrot, finely chopped

½ cucumber, peeled and finely chopped

½ red pepper, deseeded and finely chopped

1tbsp tamari

Blend the parsnips and tahini in a high-powered blender. Add the tahini parsnip mixture to the sheets of nori. Top the mixture with the rest of the vegetables and drizzle with tamari. Roll and enjoy.

♥ ♥ ♥

Mexican Chili
Serves 2

1tbsp olive oil

1 red onion, sliced

2 garlic cloves, peeled and crushed

½ red pepper, deseeded and sliced

½tsp chili powder

1tsp paprika

1tsp ground cumin

1tsp ground coriander (cilantro)

1tbsp tamari

400g (14oz) can of chopped tomatoes

1tbsp tomato puree

400g (14oz) can of red kidney beans, drained and rinsed

2tsp xylitol

2 handfuls beansprouts

1 spring onion (scallion), finely chopped

Heat the olive oil in a large pan and gently sauté the onion, garlic, pepper, chili, paprika, cumin, coriander, and tamari. Cover and steam fry over a low heat for 5 minutes. Add the chopped tomatoes, tomato puree, kidney beans, and xylitol and cook for a further 15–20 minutes, stirring occasionally to prevent it sticking. Add a little water if the mixture becomes too thick, and cook until the vegetables are just tender. Garnish with beansprouts and spring onion, and serve with a large salad.

❤ ❤ ❤

Peace Pots
Serves 2

100g (4oz) uncooked quinoa

240ml (8fl oz) vegetable stock (yeast-free stock cube)

400g (14oz) can of chickpeas, drained and rinsed

2 cabbage leaves, finely chopped

2 carrots, grated

2 handfuls beansprouts

1 red onion, finely chopped

8 shitake mushrooms, finely chopped

For the dressing:

1tbsp fresh coriander (cilantro), finely chopped

2tbsps tamari

1tbsp maple syrup/agave nectar/1 sachet of stevia

Cook the quinoa in the vegetable stock according to the packet instructions. Combine the chickpeas, cabbage, carrots, beansprouts, onion, and shitake mushrooms. Place half the quinoa in the bottom of each bowl and top with the mixed vegetables. For the dressing, mix the coriander, tamari, and maple syrup. Pour the dressing over the top of the vegetables and serve.

❤ ❤ ❤

Hot Smoking Potato
Serves 1

1 large sweet potato

1dsp dairy butter

Pinch of paprika

Pinch of sea salt (to taste)

Place the whole sweet potato in a pre-heated oven at 220°C (425°F) Gas Mark 7 for 45 minutes or until soft. Remove, cut open, fill with the butter and paprika, and season with sea salt. Serve with a large green salad.

❤ ❤ ❤

Posh Quinoa
Serves 2

1tbsp olive or coconut oil

2 garlic cloves, peeled and minced

1 red onion, finely chopped

2.5cm (1in) root ginger, peeled and minced

1 red pepper, deseeded and finely chopped

8 shitake mushrooms, finely chopped

1 carrot, finely chopped

400ml (14fl oz) yeast-free vegetable stock (stock cube)

400g (14oz) uncooked quinoa

1tbsp fresh, chopped coriander (cilantro)

2tbsps tamari

Mixed herbs and sea salt to season (to taste)

Heat the oil in a pan and sauté the garlic, onion, and ginger for 2–3 minutes. Add the pepper, mushrooms and carrot and cook for a further 5 minutes. Add the vegetable stock and quinoa and simmer for 10 minutes until quinoa is tender but not mushy. Add more water if needed. Mix in the coriander and tamari, and season to taste. Enjoy hot or cold.

♥♥♥

Mineral Rich Nori Omelet
Serves 1

4 free-range eggs

½ red pepper, finely chopped

1 small red onion, finely chopped

4 shitake mushrooms, chopped

1 nori sheet, crushed

1tsp dairy butter

Whisk the eggs in a bowl. Add the pepper, onion, mushrooms, and nori. Melt the butter over a medium heat, add the mixture and cook until the egg becomes semi firm. Fold and cook until the egg is firm.

♥♥♥

Tomato and Balsamic Baked Cod
Serves 2

2 cod fillets

6 cherry tomatoes

1 red onion, finely chopped

1 tsbp basil, finely chopped

1 clove garlic, finely chopped

1 tbsp balsamic vinegar

1 tbsp olive oil

Sea salt to season

Place all the ingredients in foil and wrap into loose parcels. Bake in a preheated oven at 220°C (425°F) Gas Mark 7 for 20 minutes. Serve with lots of green leafy, or non-starchy, vegetables.

♥♥♥

Quinoa Kedgeree
Serves 2

100g (4oz) uncooked quinoa

240ml (8fl oz) vegetable stock (yeast-free stock cube)

2 fillets line-caught haddock

1 onion, chopped

1 clove garlic, minced

150g (5oz) frozen peas

1 tsp olive oil

2 organic, free-range eggs, hard boiled, peeled and chopped

480ml (16fl oz) dairy-free milk

2 tsp of curry powder

1 tbsp fresh coriander (cilantro), chopped

Sea salt to taste

Poach the haddock in the milk for a couple of minutes until cooked. Sauté the onion and garlic in the olive oil for a couple of minutes. Flake the fish into chunks and, with the milk, combine it with the onion and garlic. Add all remaining ingredients and heat the mixture gently until the peas are heated through, adding more milk if required.

♥♥♥

Desserts

Cashew Cream
Serves 2

400g (14oz) soaked cashew nuts

240ml (8fl oz) nondairy coconut milk or nut milk (not tinned coconut milk!)

120ml (4fl oz) agave nectar/maple syrup (add more for sweetness)

Soak the cashews in enough water to cover for 3–4 hours and drain. Add to a high-powered blender. Slowly add some coconut milk and the agave nectar. You can keep the mixture thick so it has the consistency of double cream or add more coconut milk to make it runnier, like single cream. For more sweetness just add more agave nectar. It should be smooth and tasty.

❤ ❤ ❤

Baked Apple Warmer
Serves 2

2 apples, sliced thinly

¼tsp ground cinnamon

¼tsp ground nutmeg

2tbsps maple syrup/agave nectar

1tsp vanilla extract

1 dollop Cashew Cream (see page 260)

Spread out the apple slices on a baking tray. Whisk together the cinnamon, nutmeg, maple syrup, and vanilla extract in a small bowl. Pour the mixture onto the apples. This dessert can be eaten raw or placed in a preheated oven at 200°C (400°F) Gas Mark 6 for 5 minutes. The flavor becomes more intense the longer the mixture is left on the apples (that is, if you can resist eating it all straight away!). Top with a dollop of Cashew Cream.

❤ ❤ ❤

Banana Whip
Serves 1

3 bananas, frozen (remove skins before freezing)

Place the bananas in a high-powered blender for 2½ minutes. Shake the mixture back down and blend for a further 2½ minutes, or until it has the consistency of creamy, soft ice cream. Serve immediately.

♥♥♥

Himalayan-salted Popcorn
Serves 1

2tbsp dairy butter/coconut oil

150g (5oz) popcorn kernels

Pinch of Himalayan/Celtic sea salt to taste

Place half the butter or coconut oil in a large pan (you'll need the lid, too) and heat for 3–4 minutes. Add the rest of the butter and the popcorn kernels. Replace the lid, reduce the heat and wait for the popping to start. Once it's finished the popcorn should be soft and chewy. Sprinkle with Himalayan sea salt and serve.

♥♥♥

Bliss Bombs
Makes 6

2tbsps hazelnut butter

1tbsp cacao powder

120ml (4fl oz) agave nectar/maple syrup

1tsp maca powder

1tbsp shredded coconut (plus additional 1–2tbsps for rolling)

Combine all the ingredients, roll into balls and then roll in extra coconut. Place in the freezer for 1 hour or until firm.

Christy's Secret Raw Chocolate
Makes 6–8 servings

240ml (8fl oz) coconut oil, melted

150g (5oz) cacao powder

60ml (2fl oz) water

120ml (4fl oz) agave nectar

120ml (4fl oz) cocoa butter, melted

1tbsp hazelnut/almond butter

Mix all the ingredients together in a bowl and pour into an ice cube tray or chocolate mold. Set in the freezer for 1 hour or until firm.

♥ ♥ ♥

Tropicana Sorbet
Serves 2

1 whole pineapple

1 dsp maple syrup (if required)

Peel and chop the pineapple into small chunks, and freeze in a plastic container for a couple of hours. Once frozen, place the pineapple in a blender with the sweetener and whiz until smooth. Serve immediately.

♥ ♥ ♥

Final Farewell

Hot, Healthy, Happy Ever After

Some days my skin declares war. Some days my adrenals freak out. Some days I stay in my PJs and eat granola from morning till night. I'm not perfect. So if you catch me throwing shapes in my stilettos with a bottle of Champagne in my hand, come and join me. If you spot me in whole foods and I'm gorging on chocolate, I'll be happy to share. Life's fun, it's messy, it's unexpected. Love it. Live it. Enjoy it.

Now that you have lived the HHH way for 21 days, do you really want to go back to how life was before? Of course not! It's onward and upward from here on. Now is the time to spread your wings. If you've found taking certain foods out of your diet difficult, then you could slowly add healthier versions back in (organic, free-range, and junk-free are the key words to remember), and see how your body responds. Take it slow and see how you go. If old symptoms return, you will know a gentle way to refresh and restart. Aim to keep around 80–90 percent of your daily routine consistent, and you will get away with the odd steak, cocktail, and cupcake every now and then. Be a portion princess, and stay hot, healthy, happy. I know you can do it.

They say that all great things come to an end, but when do we listen to what everyone else says? Let's keep this party going! It may be the end of the book but your hot, healthy, happy journey isn't over. Come and visit me at www.thefoodpsychologist.com. I have some special surprises up my virtual sleeve and you won't want to miss them. I'd love to hear how you got on with the HHH 21-day diet. If you want to send me an e-mail or video testimonial, I would be absolutely over the moon, so please get typing or recording. If you want some airplay then include a link to your site, Twitter, or Facebook page because I love sharing great stories.

Want to spread the love and help others get hot, healthy, happy, too? Way to go, girl! This is a movement. We're recruiting. We need numbers. We need fabulous you. So share this book. Tweet out your love with @DrChristyPhD in your message. E-mail your whole contact list if you feel so inspired. Rave about *Hot, Healthy, Happy* on Facebook. Review it online or on your site. Tell your friends that science makes them sexy, hold up this book, and give a cheeky little wink. They'll catch your drift. Make hot, healthy, happy a trend. Up for it? Fabulous! Use the hashtag #hothealthyhappy.

See you soon, hot stuff!

Love, Christy x

Endnotes

Part I

Chapter 1: Let's Get Personal

1. 'What is functional medicine?' The Institute of Functional Medicine http://www.functionalmedicine.org/about/whatisfm/ [accessed January 7, 2013]

Chapter 2: What They Don't Want You To Know

1. Cousens, G. *Conscious Eating* (North Atlantic Books, 2000)

2. Denoon, D.J. 'Drink more soda gain more weight?'; http://www. webmd.com/diet/news/20050613/drink-more-diet-soda-gain-more-weight [accessed October 1, 2012]

3. Mindell, E.L. and Hopkins, V. *Prescription Alternatives* (Bottom Line, 2003)

4. Blaylock, R.L. *Excitotoxins, the Taste that Kills* (Health Press, 1997)

Part II

Chapter 1: Eat Yourself Skinny

1. Bozarth, M.A. 'Pleasure systems in the brain,' in Warburton D.M. (ed.), *Pleasure: The Politics and the Reality* (John Wiley & Sons, 1994; 5–14)

2. Oettle, G. *et al.* 'Glucose and insulin responses to manufactured and whole-food snacks,' *Am J Clin Nutr* 1987; 45: 86–91

3. Koh, K. *et al.* 'The hunger-obesity paradox: obesity in the homeless,' Journal of Urban Health cited in Keim B. 'Homeless and overweight: obesity is the new malnutrition' (June 4, 2012); *http://www.wired.com/wiredscience/2012/06/homeless-obesity/* [accessed December 1, 2012]

4. Scheirer, L.M. 'What is the hunger-obesity paradox?' *J Am Diet Assoc.* 2005; 105(6): 883–4

5. Monteiro, C. *et al.* 'Increasing consumption of ultra-processed foods and likely impact on human health: Evidence from Brazil,' *Public Health Nutrition* 2011; 14(1): 5–13

6. Song, Q. *et al.* 'Processed food consumption and risk of esophageal squamous cell carcinoma: A case-control study in the high risk area,' Cancer Science cited by Poliquin Editorial Staff, 'Seven reasons to eliminate processed food from your diet in favour of whole foods' (August 21, 2012); *http://www.charlespoliquin.com/ArticlesMultimedia/Articles/Article/919/Seven_Reasons_to_Eliminate_Processed_Foods_from_Yo.aspx* [accessed December 1, 2012]

7. Fretts, A. *et al.* 'Associations of processed meat and unprocessed red meat intake with incident diabetes: The strong heart family study,' *Am J Clin Nutr* 2012; 95(3): 752–8

8. Olney, J.W. *et al.* 'Increasing brain tumor rates: Is there a link to aspartame?' *J. Neuropathol Exp Neurol* 1996; 55: 1115–23

9. Weinbrauch, M.R, and Diehl, V. 'Artificial sweeteners – do they bear a carcinogenic risk,' *Ann Oncol* 2004; 15(10): 1460–5

10. Sejersted, O.M. *et al.* 'Format concentrations in plasma from patients poisoned with methanol,' Acta Med Scand. 1983; 213: 105–10 cited by Mercola, J. 'Artificial sweeteners – more dangerous than you ever imagined' (October 13, 2009); *http://articles.mercola.com/sites/articles/archive/2009/10/13/artificial-sweeteners-more-dangerous-than-you-ever-imagined.aspx#_ednref10* [accessed December 1, 2012]

11. Olney, J.W. *et al.* 'Increasing brain tumor rates: Is there a link to aspartame?' *J. Neuropathol Exp Neurol* 1996; 55: 1115–123

12. He, K. *et al.* 'Consumption of monosodium glutamate in relation to incidence of overweight in Chinese adults: China health and nutrition survey (CHNS)' *Am J Clin Nutr* 2011; 93(6): 1328–1336

13. He, K. *et al.* 'Association of monosodium glutamate intake with overweight in Chinese adults: the INTERMAP Study,' *Obesity* 2008; 16(8): 1875–80

14. Braylock, R. 'Dr. Blaylock: MSG can make you fat – and sick,' Newsmax Health 2011; http://www.newsmaxhealth.com/headline_health/Blaylock_MSG_Obesity/2011/06/07/392446.html [accessed October 1, 2012]

15. 'Truth labeling collected reports of adverse reactions caused by MSG'; http://www.truthinlabeling.org/adversereactions.html [accessed October 1, 2012]

16. 'Names of Ingredients that contain processed free glutamic acid (MSG)'; http://www.truthinlabeling.org/hiddensources.html [accessed October 1, 2012]

17. Chajes, V. *et al.* 'Association between serum trans-monounsaturated fatty acids and breast cancer risk in E3N-EPIC study,' *Am J Epidemiol* 2008; 167: 1312–20

18. Mozaffarian, D. *et al.* 'Trans fatty acids and cardiovascular disease,' *N Engl J Med* 2006; 354: 1601–13

19. Sanborn, M. *et al.* 'Pesticides literature review,' Ontario College of Family Physicians 2004; http://www.ocfp.on.ca/docs/public-policy-documents/pesticides-literature-review.pdf [accessed October 1, 2012]

20. Jakszyn, P. and Gonzalez, C.A. 'Nitrosamine and related food intake and gastric and esophageal cancer risk: A systematic review of the epidemiological evidence,' *World Journal of Gastroenterology* 2006; 12 (27): 4296–303

21. Heini A.F. and Weinsier, R.L. 'Divergent trends in obesity and fat intake patterns: The American paradox' *Am J Med*. 1997; 102(3): 259–64

22. Abbatecola, A.M. *et al.* 'Insulin resistance and executive dysfunction in older persons,' *Journal of American Geriatric Society* 2004; 52(10): 1713–18

23. Moore, S.C. 'Violence and society research group, applied clinical research,' *Br J Psychiatry* 2009; 195: 366–7

24. Whitney, E.N. and Rolfes, S.R. *Understanding Nutrition* (Wadsworth Centre of Learning, 2009)

25. Salmeron, J. *et al.* 'Dietary fiber, glycemic load, and risk of non-insulin-dependent diabetes mellitus in women,' *JAMA* 1997; 277(6): 472–7

26. Dong, J. *et al.* Dietary glycemic index and glycemic load in relation to the risk of type 2 diabetes: a meta-analysis of prospective cohort studies, *Br J Nutr* 2011; 106(11): 1649–54

27. Barclay, A.W. *et al.* 'Glycemic index, glycemic load, and chronic disease risk: A meta-analysis of observational studies,' *Am J Clin Nutr* 2008; 87(3): 627–37

28. Krone, C.A. and Ely, J.T. 'Controlling hyperglycemia as an adjunct to cancer therapy,' *Integrative Cancer Therapies* 2005; 4(1): 25–31

29. Thomas, D.E. *et al.* 'Low glycemic index or low glycemic load diets for overweight and obesity,' *Cochrane Database of Systematic Reviews*, 2007; Issue 3

30. Pereira, M.A. *et al.* 'Effects of a low-glycemic load diet on resting energy expenditure and heart disease risk factors during weight loss,' *JAMA* 2004; 292: 2482–90

31. Ludwig, D. 'The glycemic index physiological mechanism relating to obesity, diabetes, and cardiovascular disease,' *JAMA* 2002; 287(18): 2414–23

32. Hyman, M. 'Gluten: What you don't know might kill you,' Huffington Post 2010; http://www.huffingtonpost.com/dr-mark-hyman/gluten-what-you-don't-know_B_379089.html [accessed October 1, 2012]

33. Sedghizadeh, P.P. *et al.* 'Celiac disease and recurrent aphthous stomatitis: a report and review of the literature,' *Oral Surg Oral Med Oral Pathol Oral Radiol Endod* 2002; 94(4): 474–8

34. Ludvigsson, J.F. *et al.* 'Coeliac Disease and Risk of Mood Disorders – a General Population-based Cohort Study,' *J Affect Disord* 2007; 99(1-3): 117–26

35. Hu, W.T. *et al.* 'Cognitive impairment and celiac disease,' *Arch Neurol* 2006; 63(10): 1440–6

36. Bushara, K.O. 'Neurologic presentation of celiac disease,' *Gastroenterology* 2005; 128(4 Suppl 1): S92-7

37. Farrell, R.J. and Kelly, C.P. 'Celiac spruce,' *N Engl J Med* 2002; 346(3): 180–8

38. Ludvigsson, J.F. *et al.* 'Small-intestinal histopathology and mortality risk in celiac disease,' *JAMA.* 2009; 302(11): 1171–8

39. Hyman, M. 'Three hidden ways gluten makes you fat,' Huffington Post 2012; wheat-gluten_B_1274872html [accessed October 1, 2012]

40. Sapone, A. *et al.* 'Spectrum of gluten-related disorders consensus on nomenclature and classification,' *BC Medicine* 2002; 10(13)

41. Katz, K.D. *et al.* 'Intestinal permeability in patients with Crohn's disease and their healthy relatives,' *Gastroenterology* 1989; 97(4): 927–31

42. Fasano A. 'Physiological, pathological, and therapeutic implications of Zonulin-medicated intestinal barrier modulation: Living life on the edge of the wall.' *Am J Pathol* 2008; 173(5): 1243–52

43. Drago, S. *et al.* 'Gliadin, zonulin and gut permeability: Effects on celiac and non-celiac intestinal mucosa and intestinal cell lines,' Scand J *Gastroenterol* 2006; 41(4): 408–19

44. Pearson, A.D. *et al.* 'Intestinal permeability in children with Crohn's disease and coeliac disease,' *Br Med J* 1982; 285(6334): 20–1

45. Pironi, L. *et al.* 'Relationship between intestinal permeability to [51Cr] EDTA and inflammatory activity in asymptomatic patients with Crohn's disease,' *Dig Dis Sci* 1990; 35(5): 582–8

46. Munkholm, P. *et al.* 'Intestinal permeability in patients with Crohn's disease and ulcerative colitis and their first degree relatives,' Gut 1994; 35(1): 68–72

47. Hollander, D. *et al.* 'Increased intestinal permeability in patients with Crohn's disease and their relatives. A possible etiologic factor,' *Ann Intern Med* 1986; 105(6): 883–5

48. Teahon, K. *et al.* 'Intestinal permeability in patients with Crohn's disease and their first degree relatives,' *Gut* 1992; 33(3): p. 320–3

49. Buret, A.G. 'Pathophysiology of enteric infections with Giardia duodenalius' *Parasite* 2008; 15(3): 261–5

50. Hamilton, I. *et al.* 'Small intestinal permeability in dermatological disease,' *Q J Med* 1985; 56(221): 559–67

51. Klee, W.A. *et al.* 'Opioid peptides derived from food proteins. The Exorphins in endorphins in mental health research,' *J Biochemical Chemistry* 1978; 254(7): 2446–9

Chapter 2: Eat Yourself Happy: Turning Dark Moods Technicolor

1. Peirson, A.R. and Heuchert, J.W. 'Correlations for serotonin levels and measures of mood in a nonclinical sample,' *Psychol Rep* 2000; 87(3 Pt 1): 707–16

2. Audhya, T. 'Advances in measurement of platet catecholamines at sub-picamole levels from diagnosis of depression and anxiety,' *Clinical Chemistry* 2005; 51(6); supplement E. 128

3. Praschak-Reider, N. et al 'Seasonal variation in human brain serotonin transporter binding FREE,' *Arch Gen Psychiatry* 2008; 65(9): 1072–8

4. Ross, J. *The Mood Cure* (Thorsons, 2002)

5. Jepson, T.L. *et al.* 'Current perspective on the management of seasonal affective disorder,' *J AM Pharm Assoc.* 39(6): 822–9

6. Even, C. *et al.* 'Efficacy of light therapy in non-seasonal depression: A systematic review,' *J Affect Disord.* 2008; 108(1–2): 11–23

7. Golden, R.N. *et al.* 'The efficacy of light therapy in the treatment of mood disorders: a review and meta-analysis of the evidence,' *Am J Psychiatry* 2005; 162(4): 656–62

8. Lyons, P.M. and Truswell, A.S. 'Serotonin precursor influenced by type of carbohydrate meal in healthy adults,' *Am J Clin Nutr* 1988; 47(3): 433–9

9. Wurtman, R. J. and Wurtman, J. J. 'Brain serotonin, carbohydrate-craving, obesity and depression,' *Obesity Research* 1995; 3: 477S–80S

10. Braverman, E.R. *The Healing Nutrients Within* (Basic Health Publishing, 2003)

11. Wurtman, R.J. 'Carbohydrate craving. Relationship between carbohydrate intake and disorders of mood,' *Drugs* 1990; 39(3): 49–52

12. Wurtman, R.J. 'Depression and weight gain: the serotonin connection.' *J Affect Disord* 1993; 29(2-3): 183–92

13. Braverman, E.R. *The Edge Effect* (Collins and Brown Limited, 2003)

14. '5-HTP: uses, side effects, interactions and warnings,' WebMD; archived from the original November 16, 2009

15. Turner, E.H. and Blackwell, A.D. '5-Hydroxytryptophan plus SSRIs for interferon-induced depression: Synergistic mechanisms for normalizing synaptic serotonin,' *Medical Hypotheses* 2005; 65(1): 138–44

16. Holford, P. *How To Quit Without Feeling Sh**t* (Piatkus, 2008)

17. Purves, D. *et al. Neuroscience* (Sinauer Associates, 2008; 4th edition: 137–8)

18. Divi, R.L. *et al.* 'Anti-thyroid isoflavones from soybean: isolation, characterization and mechanism of action,' *Biochem Pharmacol* 1997; 15; 54(101): 1087–96

19. Young, S. N. 'How to increase serotonin in the human brain without drugs,' *J Psychiatry Neurosci.* 2007; 32(6): 394–9

20. Hao, S. *et al.* 'Separation-induced body weight loss, impairment in alternation behavior, and autonomic tone effects of tyrosine,' *Pharmacol Biochem. Behav* 2001; 68(2): 273–81

21. Magill, R.A. *et al.* 'Effects of tyrosine, phentermine, caffeine D-amphetamine, and placebo on cognitive and motor performance deficits during sleep deprivation,' *Nutritional Neuroscience* 2003; 6 (4): 237–46

22. Neri, D.F. *et al.* 'The effects of tyrosine on cognitive performance during extended wakefulness,' *Aviation, Space, and Environmental Medicine* 1995; 66(4): 313–9

23. Reinstein, D.K., *et al.* 'Dietary tyrosine suppresses the rise in plasma corticosterone following acute stress in rats,' *Life Sci.* 1985; 37(23): 2157–63

24. Klee, W.A. *et al.* 'Opioid peptides derived from food proteins. The exorphins in endorphins in mental health research,' *J. Biochemical Chemistry* 1978; 254(7): 2446–9

25. Cooper, J.R. *et al. The Biochemical Basis of Neurophamacology* (Oxford University Press, 1996: 431–2)

26. Klee, W.A. *et al.* 'Opioid peptides derived from food proteins. THE EXORPHINS in endorphins in mental health research,' *J Biochemical Chemistry* 1978; 254(7): 2446–9

27. Barnard, N. *The 21-Day Weight Loss Kick Start Diet* (Headline, 2011: 159)

Chapter 3: Do You Have the Guts to be Healthy

28. Lo, C.C. *et al.* 'Implication of anti-parietal cell antibodies and anti-helicobacter pylori,' *World Journal of Gastroenterology* 2005; 11(30): 4715–20

29. Skikne, B.S., Lynch, S.R., Cook, J.D. 'Role of gastric acid in food iron absorption,' *Gastroenterology* 1981; 81:1068–70

30. Recker, R.R. ' Calcium absorption and achlorhydria,' *New Engl J Med* 1985; 313(2): 70–3

31. Krasinski, S.D. *et al.* 'Fundic atrophic gastritis in an elderly population: effect on hemoglobin and several serum nutritional indicators,' *Journal of American Geriatrics* 1986; 34: SOO–6

32. Periera, R.S. 'Regression of gastroesophageal reflux disease symptoms using dietary supplementation with melatonin, vitamins and amino acids: Comparison with omeprazole,' *J Pineal Res.* 2006; 41(3): 195–200

33. Wilson, J.L. *Adrenal Fatigue: The 21st Century Stress Syndrome* (Smart Publications, 2001)

34. Rolfe, R.D. 'The role of probiotic cultures n the control of gastro-intestinal health,' *Journal of Nutrition* 2001; 130: 3965–4025

35. Elmer, G.W. 'Probiotics: living drugs,' *American Journal of Health-Systems, Pharmacy* 2001, 58(12): 1101–9

36. Wang, X. and Gibson, G.R. Effects of the in vitro fermentation of oligofructose and inulin by bacteria growing in the human large intestine,' *J Applied Bacteriol* 1993; 75: 373–80

37. Dodd, H.M. and Gasson, M.J. *Genetics & Biotech of Lactic Acid Bacteria* (Blackie & Sons, 1994: 211–51)

38. Roberfroid, M. J. 'Concepts of functional foods: The case of inulin and oligofructose,' *Nutrition* 1999; 129(7): 1398S–1401S

39. Wang, X. and Gibson, G.R. 'Effects of the in vitro fermentation of oligofructose and inulin by bacteria growing in the human large intestine,' *J Applied Bacteriol* 1993; 75: 373–80

40. Pearson, A.D. *et al.* 'Intestinal permeability in children with Crohn's disease and coeliac disease,' *Br Med J* 1982; 285(6334): 20–1

41. Pironi, L. *et al.* 'Relationship between intestinal permeability to [51Cr] EDTA and inflammatory activity in asymptomatic patients with Crohn's disease,' *Dig Dis Sci* 1990; 35(5): 582–8

42. Munkholm, P. *et al.* 'Intestinal permeability in patients with Crohn's disease and ulcerative colitis and their first degree relatives,' *Gut* 1994; 35(1): 68–72

43. Hollander, D. *et al.* 'Increased intestinal permeability in patients with Crohn's disease and their relatives. A possible etiologic factor,' *Ann Intern Med* 1986; 105(6): 883–5

44. Teahon, K. *et al.* 'Intestinal permeability in patients with Crohn's disease and their first degree relatives,' *Gut* 1992; 33(3): 320–3

45. Buret, A.G. 'Pathophysiology of enteric infections with giardia duodenalius,' *Parasite* 2008; 15(3): 261–5

46. Hamilton, I. *et al.* 'Small intestinal permeability in dermatological disease,' *Q J Med* 1985; 56(221): 559–67

47. Cariello, R. *et al.* 'Intestinal permeability in patients with chronic liver diseases: Its relationship with the aetiology and the entity of liver damage,' *Dig Liver Dis* 2010; 42(3): 200–4

48. Mack, D.R. *et al.* 'Correlation of intestinal lactulose permeability with exocrine pancreatic dysfunction,' *J Pediatr* 1992; 120: 696–701

49. Jalonen, T.J. 'Identical intestinal permeability changes in children with different clinical manifestations of cow's milk allergy,' *Allergy Clin Immunol* 1991; 88(5): 737–42

50. Barau, E. and Dupont, C. 'Modifications of intestinal permeability during food provocation procedures in pediatric irritable bowel syndrome,' *J Pediatr Gastroenterol Nutr* 1990; 11(1): 72–7

51. Paganelli, R. *et al.* 'Intestinal permeability in irritable bowel syndrome. Effect of diet and sodium cromoglycate,' *Ann Allergy* 1990; 64(4): p. 377–80

52. Brun, P. *et al.* 'Increased intestinal permeability in obese mice: new evidence in the pathogenesis of nonalcoholic steatohepatitis,' *Am J Physiol Gastrointest Liver Physiol* 2007; 292(2): 518–25

53. Cani P.D. *et al.* 'Changes in gut microbiota control inflammation in obese mice through a mechanism involving GLP-2-driven improvement of gut permeability,' *Gut* 2009; 58(8): 1091–103

54. Clayton, P. *Health Defence* (Accelerated Learning Systems, 2nd Ed., 2004)

55. Wang, X. and Gibson, G.R. 'Effects of the in vitro fermentation of oligofructose and inulin by bacteria growing in the human large intestine,' *J Applied Bacteriol* 1993; 75: 373–80

56. Peng, X. *et al.* 'Effects of enteral supplementation with glutamine granules on intestinal mucosal barrier function in severe burned patients,' *Burns* 2004; 30(2): 135–9

Chapter 4: Hormonal Havoc: Managing Your Monthly Madness

1. Woolans, C. *Oestrogen The Killer in Our Midst* (Health Issues Ltd, 2004)

2. Newbold, R.R. *et al.* 'Developmental exposure to endocrine disruptors and the obesity epidemic,' *Reproductive Toxicology* 2007; 23(3): 290–6

3. Lee, J. Natural *Progesterone: the Multiple Roles of a Remarkable Hormone* (BLL Publishing, 1993: 42)

4. Caulifield, L. *et al.* 'Potential contribution of maternal zinc supplementation during pregnancy to maternal and child survival,' *Am J Clin Nutr* 1998; 68: 499S–508S

5. Hays, B. 'Female hormones: the dance of the hormone, part 1' in Jones, D. (ed.), *The Textbook of Functional Medicine* (Institute of Functional Medicine, 2005)

6. Kaaks, R. *et al.* 'Postmenopausal serum androgens, oestrogens and breast cancer risk: The European prospective investigation into cancer and nutrition,' *Endocrine-Related Cancer* 2005; 12 (4): 1071–82

7. McArdle, O. and O'Mahoney, D. *Oncology: An Illustrated Color Text* (Elsevier, 2008)

8. Bulun, S.E. 'Endometriosis,' *New Engl J Med* 2009; 360(3): 268–79

9. Ross, R.K. *et al.* 'Risk Factors for uterine fibroids. Reduced risk associated with oral contraceptive,' *BMJ* (Clinical Res Ed) 1986; 293: 359–62

10. Wardle, P. and Fox, R. 'Symptoms of oestrogen deficiency in women with oestrodial implants,' *BMJ* 1989; 299: 1102

11. Neil, K. and Holford, P. *Balancing Hormones Naturally* (Piatkus, 1998)

12. Neil, K. 'Sex imbalances,' in Nicolle, L. and Woodriff Beirne, A. (ed.) *Biochemical Imbalances in Disease* (Singing Dragon, 2010)

13. 'Combined contraceptive pill side effects NHS,' in NHS, 2012; http://www.nhs.uk/Conditions/Combined-contraceptive-pill/Pages/Side-effects.aspx [accessed October, 1 2012]

14. Franceschi, S. 'The IARC commitment to cancer prevention: The example of papillomavirus and cervical cancer,' *Recent Results in Cancer Research* 2005; 166: 277–97

15. Hunter, D.J. *et al.* 'Oral contraceptive use and breast cancer: A prospective study of young women,' *Cancer Epidemiol Biomarkers Prev* 2010; 19(10): 2496–502

16. Collaborative Group on Hormonal Factors in Breast Cancer, 'Breast cancer and hormonal contraceptives: collaborative reanalysis of individual data on 53 297 women with breast cancer and 100 239 women without breast cancer from 54 epidemiological studies,' *Lancet* 1996; 22; 347(9017): 1713–27

17. Scholes, D. *et al.* 'Oral contraceptive use and bone density change in adolescent and young adult women: a prospective study of age, hormone dose, and discontinuation,' *Journal of Clinical Endocrinology & Metabolism* 2011; 10(1210): 2010–3027

18. Roberts, S.C. *et al.* 'MHC-correlated odour preferences in humans and the use of oral contraceptives.' Proceedings,' *Biological Sciences, The Royal Society* 2008; 275 (1652), 2715–22

19. Braverman, E.R. *The Edge Effect* (Collins and Brown Limited, 2003)

20. Hankinson, S.E. *et al.* 'Circulating concentrations of insulin-like growth factor-I and risk of breast cancer,' *Lancet* 1998; 351:1393–6

21. Chan, J.M. *et al.* 'Plasma insulin-like growth factor-I and prostate cancer risk: a prospective study,' *Science* 1998; 279: 563–6

22. Diamond, H. and Diamond, M. *Fit for Life* (Bantam Paperbacks, 2004)

23. Cousens, G. *Conscious Eating* (North Atlantic Books, 2000)

24. Kurek, M. *et al.* 'A naturally occurring opioid peptide from cow's milk, beta-casomorphine-7, is a direct histamine releaser in man,' *Int Arch Allergy Immunol* 1992; 97(2): 115–20

25. Steinman, D. *Diet for a Poisoned Planet* (Thunder Mouth Press, 2006)

26. White, L.R. *et al.* 'Association of mid-life consumption of tofu with late cognitive impairment and dementia: the Honolulu-Asia aging study,' *Fifth International Conference on Alzheimer's Disease*, 27, Osaka, Japan, 1996 cited by Weston A. Price Foundation 'Soy and the brain,' 2004 [accessed October 1, 2012]

27. Allerd, C.D. *et al.* 'Soy diets containing varying amount of geinstein stimulate growth of estrogen-dependent (MCF-7) tumors in a dose-dependent manner,' *Cancer Res* 2001; 61(13): 5945–50

28. Divi, R.L. *et al.* 'Anti-thyroid isoflavones from soybean: isolation, characterization and mechanism of action,' *Biochem Pharmacol* 1997; 15 (54): 1087–96

29. Verhoeven, D.T. *et al.* 'Epidemiological studies on brassica vegetables and cancer risk,' *Cancer Epidemiol Biomarkers Prev* 1996; 5(9): 733–48

30. Zhang, Y. 'Cancer-preventive isothiocyanates: measurement of human exposure and mechanism of action,' *Mutat Res* 2004; 555(1–2): 173–90

31. Wilson, J.L. Adrenal *Fatigue: The 21st Century Stress Syndrome* (Smart Publications, 2001)

32. Okamato, Y. *et al.* 'Novel estrogenic microsomal metabolites from phthalate ester,' *Journal of Health Science* 2004; 50 (5): 556–60

Chapter 5: Beat Breakouts: The Formula for Supermodel Skin

33. Cibula, D. *et al.* 'The role of androgens in determining acne severity in adult women,' *Br J Dermatol* 2000; 143: 399–404

34. Voegeli, S.K. *et al.* 'Androgen Dependence of Hirsutism, Acne and Alopecia in Women,' *Medicine* 2009; 88: 32–45

35. Thiboutot, D. and Chen, W. 'Update and future of hormonal therapy in acne,' *Dermatology* 2003; 206: 57–67

36. Rahman, M. *et al.* Association of Serum Testosterone with Acne Vulgaris in Women,' *BSNNU* 2012; J; 5(1): 1–5

37. Zhan, H. *et al.* 'Risk factors for sebaceous gland diseases and their relationship to gastrointestinal dysfunction in Han adolescents,' *J Dermatol* 2008; 35: 555–61

38. García-Lafuente, A. *et al.* 'Derangement of mucosal barrier function by bacteria colonizing the rat colonic mucosa,' *Eur J Clin Invest* 1998; 28: 1019–26

39. Kim, J. *et al.* 'Dietary effect of lactoferrin-enriched fermented milk on skin surface lipid and clinical improvement of acne vulgaris,' *Nutrition* 1998; 26: 90

40. El-Awaki, Z. *et al.* 'Does the plasma levels of vitamin A and E affect acne condition?' *Clin Exp Dermato* 2006; 31(3): 430–4

41. Holford, P. and Savona, N. *Solve Your Skin Problems* (Piaktus, 2009)

42. Clayton, P. *Health Defence* (Accelerated Learning Systems, 2nd Ed., 2004)

43. Kaymak, Y. *et al.* 'Zinc Levels in Patients with Acne Vulgaris,' *J Turk Acad Dermatol* 2007; 1(3): 71302a

44. Rogers, S. *Detoxify or Die* (Sand Key Inc., 2002)

45. 'Cosmetics and Fragrances: Market Report Plus,' Research and Markets 2007; www.researchandmarkets.com

46. Mellowship, D. *Toxic Beauty* (Octopus Publishing Group, 2009)

Part III
Chapter 1: Think Yourself Hot, Healthy, Happy

1. Hamilton, D. *It's the Thought that Counts* (Hay House, 2006)

2. Pert, C.B. *Molecules to Emotion* (Scribner, 1997)

Part IV
Chapter 1: Ingredients for a Hot, Healthy, Happy Life

1. Pert, C.B. *Molecules to Emotion* (Scribner, 1997)

2. Carmody, R. *et al.* 'Energetic consequences of thermal and nonthermal food processing,' *Proceedings of the National Academy of Sciences* 2011; 108(48): 19199–203

3. Carmody, R. and Wrangham, R. 'The energetic significance of cooking,' *Journal of Human Evolution* 2009; 57: 379–91

4. Wiles, M.R. *et al. Essentials of Dermatology for Chiropractors*, (Jones & Bartlett Publishers, 2010).

Index

5-HTP 42, 43, 47, 50

A
acid reflux 52, 54, 75, 158
acne 79, 83–4
additives 22, 24
adrenal fatigue (burn out) 55, 74–6,
    103, 184
adrenal glands 45, 54–5, 73–6, 103
adrenalin 44, 73, 76
aflatoxins 182
alcohol 82, 88, 168, 187–8
    wine 28, 192, 208
algae 163, 185, 186, 187
alkali 155
    alkalizing nutrients/food 54, 82,
        158–60, 184, 197, 240
allergenic food 57, 157–8
almonds/almond products 43, 45,
    70, 181, 247, 248, 264
amandamide 48
amaranth 32, 49, 161, 178, 179, 197
        amino acids 42, 43, 45, 50, 82,
        180
amylopectin A 33
androgens 83–4
    see also testosterone
animal products 172
    animal fats 84
    animal protein 161, 197
anti-fungals 59, 61
antibiotics 188
antioxidants 80, 81, 82, 89, 184, 185
apple cider vinegar 53, 60, 166, 182,
    197, 210, 230–31

apples 36, 158, 176, 244, 245, 246, 262
arsenic 66
artificial flavoring 22, 172
artificial sweeteners 13, 24, 50, 58, 172
asparagus 60
aspartame 13, 22, 24, 172
attraction, law of 140–41
autoimmune diseases 14, 58, 155
avocados 36, 43, 45, 66, 84, 162, 180,
        195, 197, 216, 245, 246, 254, 255

B
bacteria 52, 56, 57, 58, 59, 83, 85, 159
    beneficial 12, 57, 60, 85, 89, 177, 182,
        187–8
baking soda baths 166
bananas 60, 176, 244, 247, 263
barley 31, 36, 158, 179
    grass 184, 185, 244, 245
bathing 78, 164, 166
beans 30, 31, 32, 36, 49, 81, 83, 177,
    194, 197
    bean soup 249–50
beansprouts 252, 258–9
beauty industry 87–8
beliefs
    bogus 132–3
    placebo effect 96–7
    toxic 94, 99, 102, 132–3
berberine 59, 61
beta-carotene 86
beta-glucuronidase 71–2
betaine 53, 59, 83
bifidobacteria 57, 188
biscuits 25

bloating 33, 34, 55, 69, 75, 157, 217
blood sugar 28–9, 30, 31, 176
    balancing 29–31, 49
    rollercoaster 21, 28, 42, 54, 75
    spikes 33, 42, 45
body brushing 165, 232
boundaries 115–26, 209
brain 38–9, 49
    and catecholamines 44–5
    and consciousness 105–6
    and endorphins 46–7
    hypothalamus 63–4
    and neuropeptides 97–8
    as a pleasure addict 42, 47–8, 49
    and polypeptides 33
    and serotonin 40–43
bran 172
bread 31, 32–3, 178
    quinoa 32
    white 27
breakfast 193–4, 248
breathing, mindful 105, 109
Brussels sprouts 72, 158
buckwheat 32, 36, 49, 161, 178, 179, 194, 197, 248, 255
bulimia 20
burn out (adrenal fatigue) 55, 74–6, 103, 184
butters 182
    nut see nut butters

C
cacao 184, 218, 245, 263, 264
cadmium 66
caffeine 13, 48, 50, 82, 168, 172, 191–2
cake 25, 32, 39, 42, 48, 99, 101, 124, 172
calcium 13, 70, 185
    calcium-d-glucarate 72
calorie-controlled diets 22
cancer 14, 22, 24, 30, 31, 68, 70
candida infections 59, 179, 188
caprylic acid 59, 61
carbohydrates
    complex 30, 36
    low-GL 30–31, 36
    refined/simple 28, 30, 42, 57, 90, 192
    and serotonin 42
carcinogens 26, 66, 72, 78, 87

carob 184
casein 48, 69, 70
caseomorphins 48
catecholamines 44–6
    see also adrenalin; dopamine
cheese 48, 172
chickpeas 177, 195, 204, 252, 253, 254, 258, 259
chicory 60
chlorine 164, 187–8
    balls 78, 164
chlorophyll 158, 159, 160, 169, 185
chocolate 39, 48, 99, 101, 124, 158, 197–8, 208, 213, 264
choline 83
chronic fatigue/chronic fatigue syndrome (CFS) 3–4, 55, 76, 80
cilantro see coriander/cilantro
coconut 162, 180
    curry 255–6
    milk 202, 247, 255, 256, 262
    nectar 179
collagen 86
colon 51, 56, 216–17
consciousness 105–9
    conscious/mindful eating 100, 102, 219
    and quantum physics 106–8
constipation 15, 51, 57, 157, 217
contraceptive pill 57, 67–8, 78, 187–8
coriander/cilantro 47, 195, 244, 245, 249, 251, 252, 253, 254, 255, 256, 257, 258–9
corn 59, 158
    see also high fructose corn syrup (HFCS)
corpus luteum 64
cortisol 54, 72, 73, 74, 75, 76, 90
cravings 35, 38, 39, 45, 48
    carbohydrate 42
    and gluten 33
    overcoming 31, 38, 48–9
crisps 25
cumin 47, 204, 256, 257, 258

D
dairy products 69, 70–71, 158, 172
    alternatives 70, 179–80
    see also specific products

depressants 168
dessert 197–8
  recipes 262–4
detergents 78, 88
detoxification 6, 58, 72, 80–83, 90
  environmental 164–5
  symptoms 166, 199, 214
  virtual 214
DHEA 55, 72, 74, 76
diabetes 13, 22, 30, 166
  type 2 14
digestion/digestive system 51–61, 75,
    77, 216–17
  digestive problems 80, 104,
      157–8, 177 see also bloating;
      constipation; indigestion
  and hormonal harmony 77, 85–6
digestive enzymes 52, 53, 56, 59, 61,
    69, 71–2, 187, 197, 217
dinner 197
  recipes 255–61
dioxins 65, 66, 82, 180
DLPA (DL-Phenylalanine) 47
DNA 95–6
dopamine 25, 44
drink 172, 183, 191–2
  herbal 36, 163, 183, 193, 208
  recipes 243–7
  soft drinks 13, 36
  water 78, 163–4
  see also juices; milkshakes;
      smoothies

E
eating
  conscious/mindful 100, 102,
      219
  emotional 99, 102, 225
  healthy see healthy eating
eggs 43, 45, 160, 172, 178
  human 64
elastin 86
emotional eating 99, 102, 225
emotional negativity 222–4
endocrine/hormone disruption 65–8,
    77, 78, 87, 88
endorphins 46–7
endotoxins 80
energy 106–8, 111, 114

enzymes 30, 158, 160, 179, 185, 196
  digestive 52, 53, 56, 59, 61, 69, 71–2,
      187, 197, 217
  P-450 81–2
EPA (eicosapentaenoic acid) 84, 163,
    185, 187
epigenetics 95–6
Epsom salts 166, 196, 230
essential fatty acids 41, 50, 159, 162,
    184, 187
estrogen 63, 64–5, 69, 71–2
  xenoestrogens 65
exercise 167, 168, 200–201, 218
exorphin 33
exotoxins 80

F
fat 26–7
  animal fats 84
  essential fatty acids 41, 50, 159, 162,
      184, 187
  and glucagon 28–9
  good quality fats 36
  and insulin 28
  in the liver 58
  raw plant fats 27, 31, 50, 84, 162–3
  saturated 82
  and sugar 27–9
  trans fats 84, 159
  and undernourishment 22
fermented food 53, 182, 230–31
fish 43, 45, 83, 158, 177–8, 197, 260–61
flavonoids 82, 185, 198, 232
flours, gluten-free 179
folic acid 54, 81, 83, 179
follicle stimulating hormone (FSH)
    64
food
  alkalizing 54, 82, 158–60, 184, 197,
      240
  allergenic 57, 157–8
  breaking up with bad food 124–5,
      171–3
  combining 161
  cravings see cravings
  dairy see dairy products
  eating see eating; healthy eating
  endorphin-boosting 47
  fermented 53, 182, 230–31

fresh/natural foods 11–12, 22–3 *see
     also* fruits; organic food; raw
     foods; vegetables
genetically modified 33
gluten-free 31–2, 34, 36, 158, 173,
     178, 179, 193–4, 196, 197, 222,
     248, 255
high-protein 45, 47, 49
industry 12–13
intolerances 31, 54, 59, 157–8
labels *see* labels, food
low-GL 30–31, 36, 73, 90, 158,
     159–60, 176
marketing 12
for the mind 109
organic *see* organic food
processed *see* processed foods
quarantine system (digestive) 52–3,
     59–60 *see also* digestion/
     digestive system
raw *see* raw foods
recipes *see* recipes
restocking for the HHH diet 173–88
serotonin-boosting 43
tyrosine-boosting 45
forgiveness 102, 226–7
formaldehyde 24
formate 24
fructooligosaccharides (FOS) 60,
     61, 85
fructose corn syrup 13
high (HFCS) 22, 25
fruits 36, 43, 165, 176
dried 176
tropical 176, 264
see also apples; bananas; oranges;
     pineapple
FSH (follicle stimulating hormone) 64
functional medicine 6–7, 237

G
gamma linoleic acid 85
garlic 59, 60, 61, 180, 195
genetically modified food 33
GI (glycemic index) 30
GL *see* glycemic load
glucagon 28–9
glucose 27–8, 30, 42, 193
glucosinolates 72

glutamine 60, 61
glutathione 81, 82
gluten 22, 31–2, 33–4, 48, 172
gluten-free food *see* food: gluten-
     free
intolerance 31, 158
gluteomorphins 33, 48
glycemic index (GI) 30
glycemic load (GL) 30
low-GL foods 30–31, 36, 73, 90, 158,
     159–60, 176
grains 30, 31, 178
granola 13, 32, 70, 178, 193, 196, 213,
     265
growth hormones 69, 76

H
HCL *see* hydrochloric acid
healing your inner child 127–38,
     223–4
healthy eating
allergen-free 157–8
breaking the rules 15
breaking up with bad food 124–5,
     171–3
conscious/mindful 100, 102, 219
and the digestive system 51–61
with fresh/natural foods 11–12,
     22–3
gluten-free *see* food: gluten-free
HHH diet *see* Hot, Healthy, Happy
     programme: 21-day diet
with high-protein foods 45, 47, 49
instinctual 14
with low GL 30–31, 36, 73, 90, 158,
     159–60, 176
and mood *see* mood
and organic food *see* organic food
overload/obsession 14–15, 98–9
pre-dinner wind down for 196
recipes for *see* recipes
slow 219
heart disease 14, 22, 31
heartburn 52, 54, 75, 158
hemp/hemp products 70, 161, 163,
     179, 180, 181, 184, 187, 195, 245,
     246, 253, 254
herbal teas 36, 163, 183, 193, 208
herbicides 165

herbs 76, 180–81, 195, 236, 244, 245
high fructose corn syrup (HFCS) 22, 25
higher self 110, 111, 118, 140, 147, 170
hormones 4, 5, 6, 50, 66, 82, 90, 160, 168
    anabolic 76 *see also* DHEA;
        growth hormones; insulin;
        testosterone
    catabolic 76 *see also* adrenalin;
        cortisol
    in dairy 69
    and digestion 77, 85–6
    growth 69, 76
    hormone/endocrine disruptors
        65–8, 77, 78, 87, 88
    hormone replacement therapy 67
    level testing 72
    sex 42, 63–78, 83–5, 88–9
    stress 45
    synthetic 67–8
    see also specific hormones
Hot, Healthy, Happy programme
    21-day diet 199–241
        and process for healthy
            digestion 59–61
    action plans
        for a healthy body 35–6, 49–50,
            61, 77–8, 89–90
        for a healthy mind 102, 113–14,
            125–6, 137–8, 149
    approach of xiii–xv, 35
    ingredients 153–70
    preparations 171–89, 191–8
    recipe suggestions *see* recipes
HRT (hormone replacement therapy)
    67
hummus 193, 194, 195, 196, 204
hunger–obesity paradox 22
hydration 163–4, 208
hydrochloric acid (HCL) 53, 54, 59–60,
    61, 89, 187, 197
hypothalamus 63–4

I
immune system 51, 58, 65–6, 73, 100,
    154, 168, 185
    autoimmune diseases 14, 58, 155
indigestion 52, 54, 75

inflammation 22
infrared saunas 87, 166–7, 201
inner child 127–38, 223–4
inner parent 129–32
insulin 27–9, 42, 76
interconnectedness 106–9, 110, 114,
    122–3
intestines 56–8, 75
    see also colon
iodine 183
iron 70

J, K
Jerusalem artichoke 60
jicama 60
juices 158, 159–60, 163
    recipes 243–4, 245–6
kimchi 182

L
labels, food 21, 22, 23, 24, 29, 164, 172,
    173–4, 177
    what they do not tell you
        13, 88
lactase 69
lactobacillus 57, 188
lactose 69
law of attraction 140–41
leaky gut 33, 58
leeks 60, 175
legumes 30, 31, 83, 177
    see also beans; peas
leptin 25
LH (luteinizing hormone) 64
liver 58, 64, 71, 80–83, 84, 86, 89
love 228
    loving yourself 100, 112–13, 122
        and your inner child 127–38,
            223–4
lucuma 184, 245
lunch 194–5
luteinizing hormone (LH) 64

M
maca 184, 238, 245, 263
magnesium 50, 68, 70, 166, 179
marine phytoplankton 185
meditation 169–70, 196

mental health/happiness
  declaring/unlocking your
      superpowers 94–5, 102, 116,
      147, 154
  and gluten 33–4
  going with the flow 110–14, 154–5
  healing your inner child 127–38,
      223–4
  and healthy boundaries 115–26
  inner chat 96
  letting go of toxic beliefs 94, 99,
      102
  and the mind–body connection
      93–102
  mindfulness see mindfulness
  positive thinking/attitude 95, 122–3
  and relaxation 101
  staying present 112–13
  and the subconscious see
      subconscious mind
  tapping into your natural power
      108
  visualizing and shaping your
      destiny 139–49
mercury 66
metabolic syndrome 22
methanol 24
methionine 83
milk 22, 69, 172
  derivatives 71
  nondairy 70, 179–80, 202, 247, 255,
      256, 262
milkshakes 183, 202, 218, 247
millet 32, 36, 49, 161, 178, 179, 197, 248
mind
  beliefs see beliefs
  coaxing the mind 142
  consciousness see consciousness
  feeding the mind 109
  and the law of attraction 140–41
  and matter 106–9, 122–3 see also
      interconnectedness
  mental health see mental health/
      happiness
  mind–body connection 93–102
  miracle-maker mindset 108–9,
      153–4
  negative thinking see negative
      thinking

positive thinking/attitude 95, 122–3
subconscious see subconscious
    mind
mindfulness 105, 109
  conscious/mindful eating 100,
      102, 219
  see also meditation
minerals 13, 30, 33, 47, 53, 54, 70, 158,
    176, 183, 185, 186, 187
  alkalizing 54
  see also specific minerals
miracle-maker mindset 108–9, 153–4
monosodium glutamate (MSG) 22, 25
mood 39–50
  and catecholamines 44–6
  and endorphins 46–7
  and serotonin 40–43
MSG (monosodium glutamate) 22, 25
muesli 248

N
negative emotions 222–4
negative patterns of behavior 220–22
negative thinking 34, 94, 104, 169
  see also beliefs: toxic
neuropeptides 97–8
neurotransmitters 39, 50
nicotine 29, 50, 73, 156
nightshades 158
nitrosamines 26
norephrine 44
nut butters 27, 70, 162, 180, 181–2, 193,
    195, 247, 252, 254, 263
nutrients 14, 27, 50, 52, 56–7, 59, 60,
    68, 72, 82, 84, 85–6, 89, 112, 154,
    156–7, 163, 185, 230
  alkalizing 54, 82, 158–60
  minerals see minerals
  nutrient deficiencies 22, 34, 35, 54, 58
  phytonutrients 66, 158, 185
  vitamins see vitamins
nuts 36, 43, 66, 84, 162, 181, 197

O
obesity–hunger paradox 22
odor preference 68
oils
  cold-pressed 66, 84, 162, 180, 187,
      195, 245, 246, 253, 254

essential 164
mineral 88
partially hydrogenated vegetable 25–6
omega fatty acids 41, 50, 159, 162, 184, 187
onions 60, 175, 194, 222
recipes with 249–61
opioid effects 33, 48
oranges 158, 169, 176
oregano 59, 61, 180, 250
organic food 23, 24, 26, 77, 83, 160, 165, 179, 185, 234
organochlorines 66
oxygen 158–9, 160, 230

P, Q
P-450 enzymes 81–2
PAH (polycyclic aromatic hydrocarbons) 66
pancreas 27, 28, 42, 52
parabens 88, 90
parents 130–32
the inner parent 129–32
partially hydrogenated vegetable oil 25–6
pasta 27, 28, 31–2, 161, 172
brown rice 194, 197, 215, 223, 239
gluten-free 34, 178
raw veggie 194
sauce 157, 215, 223, 239
pastries 48
PCBs (polychlorinated biphenyls) 66, 69
PEA (phenylethylamine) 48
peanut butter 182
peanuts 158
peas 83, 175, 261
pepsin 53, 59, 61, 187, 197
Pert, Candace 97
pesticides 25, 26, 66, 78, 87, 165
petroleum 88
phenylethylamine (PEA) 48
phosphoric acid 13
phthalates 66, 77, 88
phytic acid 70
phytonutrients 66, 158, 185
phytoplankton 185
pineapple 176, 206, 244, 264

pituitary gland 63–4, 73
placebo effect 96–7
plant tannins 59, 61
polypeptides 33
porridge 194, 248
positive thinking/attitude 95, 122–3
potatoes 158, 161, 176, 222
prebiotics 60, 61, 187–8
premenstrual syndrome (PMS) 40, 65, 75
present moment 112–13
preservatives 22, 24, 26, 157
probiotics 60, 177, 187–8
processed foods
addictiveness of 22
effect on beneficial bacteria 57
and gluten 32
nutritional deficiency of 13, 21, 22, 157
recognizing what is bad 22, 23, 24–6
saying goodbye to 172
vegetarian 161
progesterone 63, 64, 72
deficiency 74
propylene glycol 88
protein 31, 41, 49, 53–4, 59
animal 161, 197
high-protein foods 45, 47, 49
plant 49, 160
powders 184–5
see also amino acids; gluten
pulses 31, 32, 36, 49, 161, 177, 197
pumpkin seeds 163, 181, 194, 248
oil from 180, 195, 245
quantum physics 106–8
quinoa 32, 36, 49, 53–4, 70, 161, 178, 179, 197, 248, 251, 256, 258–60, 261

R
raw foods 60, 158–9, 163, 197
raw plant fats 27, 31, 50, 84, 162–3
see also fruits; salads; vegetables
rebounding 167
recipes 243–64
breakfast
Muesli, Homemade 248
Porridge, Gluten-free 248

dessert
  Baked Apple Warmer 262
  Banana Whip 263
  Bliss Bombs 263
  Cashew Cream 262
  Chocolate, Christy's Secret Raw
    264
  Popcorn, Himalayan-salted 263
  Sorbet, Tropicana 264
juice, smoothie and drink
  Almond Milk 247
  Bananarama Milkshake 247
  Ella Berry Smoothie 246–7
  Green Goddess Juice 243–4
  Green Guru 246
  Green Smoothie 244–5
  Rainbow Cocktail 246
  Sunshine Elixir 245
main course
  Coconut Curry 255–6
  Mexican Chili 257–8
  Omelet, Mineral Rich Nori 260
  Peace Pots 258–9
  Potato, Hot Smoking 259
  Quinoa, Posh 259–60
  Quinoa Kedgeree 261
  'Sushi', Rawlicious 257
  Tomato and Balsamic Baked Cod
    260–61
  Vegetable Fajitas 256–7
starter, soup and salad
  An Avocado a Day 254
  Avocado Sandwich, Open-Face
    255
  Bean Soup 249–50
  Butter Nutty Soup 250
  Chick Salad 253
  Colors of The Rainbow 251–2
  Kale and Quinoa Love Affair 253–4
  'Peanut' Satay Salad 252
  Portobello Mushrooms 250–51
  Skinny Dippers 254–5
  Vegetable Soup 249
reflux 52, 54, 75, 158
relaxation 101, 196
rice, brown 43, 178
  basmati 36
  brown rice pasta 194, 197, 215, 223,
    239

rice, white 172, 192
Ross, Julia 47
rye 31, 36, 158

S
SAD (seasonal affective disorder) 41
salads 163, 194–5, 197
  recipes 251–5
salicylate foods 158
salsolinol 48
salt 13, 74, 172, 180, 194, 240
sauerkraut 182
seasonal affective disorder (SAD) 41
seasonings 180–81
seaweed 158, 177, 182–3, 231
seeds 36, 66, 84, 163, 181, 197, 230, 245
selenium 86, 87
self-love 100, 112–13
  loving your inner child 127–38,
    223–4
self-respect 118, 119
  and boundaries 115–26
serotonin 40–43, 47, 50
  saboteurs 41, 50
sesame 163, 181, 194, 195, 248
sex hormones 42, 63–78, 83–5, 88–9
shellfish 158
skin 79–90, 165, 232
  and sunscreens 169
sleep 167–8, 223
SLS (sodium lauryl sulphate) 88, 89
smoothies 24, 159–60, 221
  recipes 244–5, 246–7
snacks 176, 183–4, 196, 220, 226
soda, diet 24
sodium lauryl sulphate (SLS) 88, 89
sodium nitrate 22, 26
soft drinks 13, 36
soup 197, 222, 228
  recipes 249–50
soya 70, 71, 158, 172, 178
spelt 31, 36
spices 47, 83, 180
spirulina 158, 161, 185, 244, 245
spreads 181–2
  nut butters see nut butters
sprouts 175, 232, 254–5
  bean 252, 258–9
  Brussels 72, 158

stevia 179, 195, 244, 252, 253, 258
stomach 52–3, 61, 216, 217, 219
    acid 53–4, 55, 57, 59, 61
    bloating see bloating
stool analysis (CDSA+P) 57, 59
stress 38, 55, 103–5, 112
    serotonin, the brain and 39, 41, 42
    stepping out of the stress response
        112–13, 114
    and tyrosine 45, 46
subconscious mind 109, 111, 141–5,
        154, 200, 221
    collective subconscious 141
    healing your inner child 127–38,
        223–4
    and the inner parent 129–32
sucralose 22, 172
sugar 21, 22, 27–9, 57, 58, 172, 192
    blood sugar see blood sugar
    glucose 27–8, 30, 42, 193
sunflower/sunflower products 24,
        163, 175, 178, 181, 194, 195, 248, 254
sunscreens 169
sunshine 40, 154, 167, 168–9, 186, 198,
        230, 234, 235
superfood powders 184–5, 200, 244,
        245
supplements 43, 45, 47, 53, 60, 61,
        84–5, 86, 185–8
    see also minerals; vitamins
sweet potatoes 32, 36, 86, 175, 194,
        197, 259
sweeteners
    artificial 13, 24, 50, 58, 172
    natural 179, 183
    sugar see sugar

T
testosterone 72, 83–4
theobromine 48
thinking see beliefs; mental health/
        happiness; mind
thrush/candida infections 59, 179,
        188

thyroid gland 45, 70, 184–5
thyroxin 72–3
time-management 211–12
toxin rehab 80–83
    see also detoxification
tryptophan 42, 43, 50
turmeric 47, 83, 180
tyrosine 45, 46, 192, 205

V
vegetables 36, 43, 45, 72, 83, 163, 165,
        175–6, 195, 197
    see also specific vegetables
visualization 108, 145–6
    creating a vision board 147–8
    and shaping your destiny 139–49
vitamins 30, 43, 47, 53, 158, 160, 176,
        185, 186
    multivitamins 186
    vitamin A 85–6, 87, 90
    vitamin B 50, 54, 81, 83, 86, 179, 185
    vitamin C 185
    vitamin D 50, 168, 169, 186
    vitamin E 87, 185

W
water 78, 163–4
    see also bathing
wheat 22, 32–4, 36, 172
wheatgrass 45, 158, 184, 244
wine 28, 192, 208

X, Y, Z
xenoestrogens 65
yacon 60, 179
yeasts 34, 57, 58, 59, 116, 155, 159
    nutritional 182
    yeast infections 55, 166
yerba mate 183, 193, 212
yo-yo dieting 19, 42, 49, 142
yoghurt 172
zinc 70, 87
zonulin 33

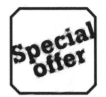
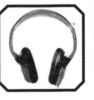
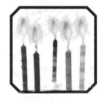
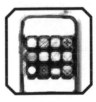
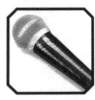
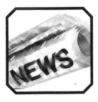
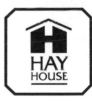

ABOUT THE AUTHOR

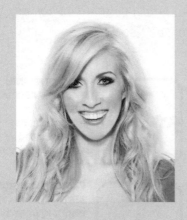

Dr. Christy Fergusson is a Doctor of Psychology, Chartered Psychologist, Nutritional Therapist, and Clinical Hypnotherapist. Known in the media as The Food Psychologist, she frequently appears as a health and nutrition expert on TV, radio, and in the press offering expert advice to help us understand our relationship with food.

Alongside her media work she runs a successful online consultancy with her husband Jonathan at www.thefoodpsychologist.com. Here she offers one-to-one coaching, online programs, and functional medicine testing to clients worldwide. She is passionate about helping others take control of their health and so offers free advice every week through her weekly online show. Her All Access Club is packed with recipes, videos, yoga, and meditation exercises designed to help empower individuals to transform their health and their bodies in a straightforward and fun way. The Food Psychologist also boasts a large online shop packed with natural beauty products, supplements, fitness and kitchen equipment, hypnotherapy and meditation downloads and more.

Christy lives in Scotland with her husband Jonathan, daughter Ella, and their two dogs Rosie and Tigger.

www.thefoodpsychologist.com